PERSONALISED MEDICINE

This book sets out a critical sociological approach to 'personalised medicine' (PM), not only highlighting its limitations and flaws but also emphasising its hopeful potentialities for a better medicine in the future.

Bringing together perspectives from science and technology studies, medical sociology, law, and bioethics, this book traces PM from its historical roots in disease classification and predictive genetics to its data-driven present of digital infrastructures, algorithmic prediction, and precision therapeutics. Across seven chapters, it explores how measurement, classification, and datafication shape medical knowledge; how infrastructures and platforms distribute benefits and risks; how publics are imagined as patients, consumers, and citizens; and how privacy, access, and equity are negotiated in global health systems. This book concludes by outlining possible futures grounded in solidarity, patient-centred care, and democratic innovation – offering practical ways to shift PM from a privilege for the few to a shared public good.

Written for scholars and practitioners in science and technology studies, sociology of medicine, health policy, and bioethics, as well as for clinicians and policymakers, this book will engage readers seeking to understand – and reshape – the social futures of data-intensive healthcare. It will also be useful for policymakers debating the implementation of different PM projects in local or national healthcare systems.

Michael Morrison is a Senior Researcher at the Centre for Health, Law and Emerging Technologies, Faculty of Law, University of Oxford. His work examines the social, ethical, and regulatory dimensions of biomedical innovation, focusing on regenerative medicine, personalised healthcare, and the governance of emerging biotechnologies.

Saheli Datta Burton is a Lecturer in Science Policy at the Department of Science and Technology Studies (UCL-STS), University College London. Her work interrogates the political-economic and governance dimensions of emerging technologies, with a focus on the geostrategic shaping of data-driven health and biomedicine.

Elisa Lievevrouw (PhD, KU Leuven) is a Postdoctoral Researcher at the Media Culture & Policy Lab, KU Leuven. She studies the interplay between innovation and policymaking in digital health and life sciences.

Elisabetta Biasin is an Associate Researcher at the KU Leuven Centre for IT & IP Law. She studies the ethical and legal aspects of healthcare technologies, with a focus on medical device, AI, cybersecurity, and data laws.

Critical Approaches to Health

Series Editors: Kerry Chamberlain & Antonia Lyons

The Routledge *Critical Approaches to Health* series aims to present critical, inter-disciplinary books around psychological, social and cultural issues related to health. Each volume in the series provides a critical approach to a particular issue or important topic, and is of interest and relevance to students and practitioners across the social sciences. The series is produced in association with the International Society of Critical Health Psychology (ISCHP).

Titles in the series:

Health Anxiety and the Quest for Safety
Interdisciplinary and Critical Perspectives
Márta Csabai

Personalised Medicine
A Critical Approach to Data-Driven Medicine
Michael Morrison and Saheli Datta Burton with Elisa Lievevrouw and Elisabetta Biasin

For more information about this series, please visit: https://www.routledge.com/Critical-Approaches-to-Health/book-series/CRITHEA

PERSONALISED MEDICINE

A Critical Approach to Data-Driven Medicine

Michael Morrison and Saheli Datta Burton

With

Elisa Lievevrouw and Elisabetta Biasin

Routledge
Taylor & Francis Group
LONDON AND NEW YORK

Designed cover image: Getty Images

First published 2026
by Routledge
4 Park Square, Milton Park, Abingdon, Oxon OX14 4RN

and by Routledge
605 Third Avenue, New York, NY 10158

Routledge is an imprint of the Taylor & Francis Group, an informa business

British Library Cataloguing-in-Publication Data
A catalogue record for this book is available from the British Library

ISBN: 9781032246314 (hbk)
ISBN: 9781032246307 (pbk)
ISBN: 9781003279556 (ebk)

DOI: 10.4324/9781003279556

Typeset in Times New Roman
by codeMantra

For Susan Kelly

CONTENTS

SERIES EDITOR PREFACE

Critical approaches to health

Health is a major issue for people all around the world and is fundamental to individual wellbeing, personal achievements, and satisfaction, as well as to families, communities, and societies. It is also embedded in social notions of participation and citizenship. Much has been written about health from a variety of perspectives and disciplines, but much of this writing takes a biomedical and positivist approach to health matters, neglecting the historical, social, and cultural contexts and environments in which health is experienced, understood, and practised. We developed this series of books to offer critical social science perspectives on important, relevant, and timely health topics.

The Critical Approaches to Health series provides new writing on health by presenting books that offer critical, interdisciplinary, and theoretical writing about health, where matters of health are framed quite broadly. The series seeks to include books ranging across important health matters, including general health-related issues (such as gender and media), major social issues for health (such as medicalisation, obesity, and palliative care), particular health concerns (such as pain, doctor–patient interaction, health services, and health technologies), particular health problems (such as diabetes, autoimmune disease, and medically unexplained illness), health for specific groups of people (such as the health of migrants, the homeless, and the aged), or combinations of these.

The series seeks above all to promote critical thought about health matters. By critical, we mean going beyond the critique of the topic and work in the field to more general considerations of power and benefit, particularly addressing concerns about whose understandings and interests are upheld, and whose are marginalised, by the approaches, findings, and practices in these various domains of health. Such critical agendas involve reflections on what constitutes knowledge, how it is created, and how it is used. Accordingly, critical approaches consider epistemological and theoretical positioning, as well as issues of methodology and practice, and seek to examine how health is enmeshed within broader social relations and structures. Books within this series take up this challenge and seek to provide new insights and understandings by applying a critical agenda to their topics. Explore the previous books in the series at https://www.routledge.com/Critical-Approaches-to-Health/book-series/CRITHEA

We are pleased to welcome the latest book in the series, *Personalised medicine: A critical approach to data-driven medicine* by Michael Morrison and Saheli Datta Burton, with co-authors Elisabetta Biasin und Elisa Lievevrouw.

This book offers a critical examination of PM, as a multifaceted and evolving set of practices that promise to transform healthcare by tailoring prevention, diagnosis, and treatment to individual biological profiles. The authors present an engaging critical sociological approach to PM, arguing that it is best understood as an ethos, an umbrella term that can be applied to a range of different technologies, projects, and practices from across medicine and healthcare. The coverage in the book is wide-ranging, documenting the many ways in which PM may be considered, and raising critical perspectives throughout. These include challenging how datafication shapes broader understandings and practices in health and medicine, and showing how the socio-technical infrastructures that underpin PM are not neutral technical arrangements but dynamic, value-laden systems with embedded visions and interests. The authors also critically discuss how the person in PM is variously imagined by science, society, and the state – as patient, consumer, citizen, beneficiary, and resister – alongside interacting imaginaries that are shaped by political, economic, and technological imperatives. The authors provide compelling arguments for how the personalisation of medicine in treatments is inherently socio-technical and political, requiring alignment between biological targeting, regulatory frameworks, and equitable healthcare delivery. And they highlight the challenges around health data governance in enabling and constraining PM, for privacy, data protection, cybersecurity, AI regulation, and sector-specific laws that govern the collection, sharing, reuse, and generation of health data.

These issues, critically developed throughout this book, are drawn together in the concluding chapter to set out a vision for a more equitable, solidaristic, and care-centred PM. In this chapter the authors propose reforms to pharmaceutical innovation, data governance, and patient engagement, so we can arrive at a human scale PM that values discretion, context, and the common good. In this way, they argue, we can ensure that data informs, but does not determine, care, and enables the sustaining of humane futures for health innovations. This is an extremely timely and important book that makes a unique, significant, and thought-provoking addition to the Critical Approaches to Health series.

In a first for the series, we are pleased to include a Foreword written by Barbara Prainsack, herself a leading researcher in the field of PM. We commend this to you for a more detailed overview, offering a thoughtful analytic commentary on both the topic of PM and the approach the authors have taken throughout this book.

Kerry Chamberlain & Antonia Lyons
November 2025

FOREWORD

by Barbara Prainsack

This book by Michael Morrison, Saheli Datta Burton, Elisabetta Biasin, and Elisa Lievevrouw offers a look at personalised medicine (PM) at a time of crisis. It is not necessarily PM that is in crisis – although, given the funding cuts in the United States and elsewhere, the beginnings of such a crisis may be in the making. What I mean by crisis here is, in the literal sense of the word, a moment of decisive change, a turning point that will define the course for the future.

In the years and months preceding the writing of this book, many assumptions and practices that had, for a long time, been part of the institutional, economic, and political landscape within which PM was set have changed. A major health emergency, COVID-19, shifted priorities and moved the so-called Overton Window. The Overton Window delineates the range of policies that are politically acceptable to publics at any given time. The COVID-19 pandemic has shifted the Overton Window by making previously unthinkable measures politically feasible, such as widespread lockdowns and other government interventions in healthcare. The pandemic led many actors to recognise the value of investing in pandemic preparedness, digital health surveillance, and public health funding beyond acute health crises. At the same time, public and political resistance to government interventions in healthcare also shifted the Overton Window in the opposite direction. They have fuelled distrust in public health institutions and led to the end of the commitment to support those that cannot pay their own way. The events in the United States in 2025, along with the statement by the chairman of the Austrian Statutory Health Insurance that healthcare need not be a 'well-equipped Mercedes' but that services at the level of a 'regular Golf' vehicle would be sufficient (Der Standard 2024), are telling manifestations of the latter development.

Against this backdrop, the authors' critical examination of various dimensions of PM could not be timelier. One of the reasons for why their examination is so fruitful lies in the authors' broad understanding of 'technologies'. Contemporary technologies of PM, the authors argue,

> include not only physical tools for sequencing genes or digital sensors for measuring heart rate and blood pressure, but also the networks of data collection, storage, and distribution, and the statistical calculations of genetic epidemiology or big data analytics that make individual measurements meaningful and medically actionable
>
> *(p5).*

This approach – which is also reflected in the focus on infrastructuring, particularly in Chapter 3 – enables the authors to examine the many subtle and less subtle ways in which PM, as a technological practice and as a governmentality, empowers and disempowers patients, families, and clinicians at the same time. This book offers new perspectives and considerations even for those familiar with PM. For example, the authors show how some of the many ways in which, next to inequities in the representation of different populations in research for PM (e.g. Johnston et al 2024; Lee 2023; Sun and Ong 2024)[1], PM can entrench or increase inequities. It does so by creating new forms of marginalisation and neglect for patients who do not have the 'right' genetic variants to receive improved treatments or products (see also Dam et al 2022)[2]. Also the high costs associated with targeted therapies and genetic testing can exacerbate inequities, both within and between countries, as healthcare budgets are strained and resources are diverted from other essential services.

One additional way in which the quest for PM can create new inequities is what I have called 'automated medicine' (Prainsack 2022). The expensive part of PM is not only cutting-edge technology but also the human experience and expertise required to interpret and 'make sense' of the data[3]. While machines may help with risk prediction and diagnosis, they cannot fully replace the judgement of human clinicians. Machine learning can identify correlations but lacks contextual understanding. In other words, although AI technologies are hailed to offer new opportunities for the automation of tasks that were previously seen as uniquely human, it is unlikely that AI will replace human ingenuity and experience completely.

This is where automated medicine comes in. Against the backdrop of current political developments in many world regions, there is a realistic chance that one of the most expensive parts of PM, namely data interpretation and other activities that require substantive input of humans, will be available only to a minority who can pay the premium for human contact. Everyone else may have to make do with the help of machines for all but the most serious and acute of health issues. As the volume of medical data grows, so does the demand for human expertise to interpret it. In regions where access to quality healthcare is limited, digital tools may seem like a viable substitute for human care. But also, in high-income countries, within healthcare systems under increasing economic strain, machine solutions may become mainstream as a 'good enough' alternative, despite their fallibility.

The groundwork for such a trend already exists. In the United States, 'boutique' or 'concierge' medicine took off in the early 2000s, when physicians started offering tailored services to a small number of patients for an annual fee (Clark et al 2011; Reinhardt 2002). By 2019, around 12,000 U.S. doctors had adopted this model, charging \$125–\$200 monthly (Daily 2019). By 2025, partly catalysed by the pandemic, the average annual membership fee had increased from \$167 to \$417 (Partner MD 2025), and the market was continually growing. Offering a combination of personalised healthcare combining high tech and high touch, boutique physicians provide same-day appointments, round-the-clock availability, and high-tech diagnostic services, including DNA sequencing. Unlike physicians in traditional fee-for-service systems, boutique doctors can spend time interpreting data with their patients, translating them into actionable information and knowledge. This ability to combine cutting-edge diagnostics with personal interaction already now, prior to the advent of automated medicine, marks a growing divide in healthcare access.

Automated medicine is what awaits us if this divide in personalisation keeps growing. Boutique medicine caters to those who can afford the monthly fees that grant them access to advanced diagnostic tests, personalised services such as annual check-ups, health coaching, and other exclusive benefits. The 99% who cannot afford this may have to suffice with automated medicine. In this model, patients would initially interact with a website or phone system, where an algorithm and chatbot gather information and provide a preliminary diagnosis. Only if their problem is deemed acute or serious enough, the patient would be directed to a first responder unit, staffed by humans. For conditions seeming non-urgent or not sufficiently serious in other regards, patients would be referred to online services for testing or monitoring. Medications would be mailed to these patients, and health monitoring would occur through apps installed on personal devices. For patients needing conversational support, a digital 'therapist' – sophisticated enough to mimic human interaction – would be assigned to assist them.

What future of personalisation do we want?

While such a scenario may seem desirable to policymakers from the perspective of cost savings, it is hardly commendable as a blueprint for a good future – and neither will it save cost in the long term. The replacement of most of the tasks of human healthcare workers by machines is likely to introduce significant hidden costs that offset or even exceed the intended savings. Patients who receive automated responses or interact primarily with AI-driven diagnostics may experience lower satisfaction, reduced trust, and decreased adherence to treatment plans, ultimately leading to worse health outcomes and increased long-term costs. The absence of human interaction can also result in more frequent errors, as machines struggle with nuance, context, and emotional cues that are crucial for effective diagnosis and care. Additionally, the burden on healthcare professionals may increase rather than decrease, as they would be required to intervene when automated systems fail or cause frustration among patients. Because AI is designed to recognise patterns and generalise from large datasets, it excels at handling standard cases. It is good at making predictions based on familiar inputs. But it struggles with outliers, because they deviate from established norms and often appear too infrequently for the model to learn how to process them effectively. Also, because AI is typically optimised for accuracy across the most common cases, rare or extreme instances are often misclassified, ignored, or dismissed as errors. This issue is compounded by AI's lack of contextual awareness – while a human expert might recognise an outlier as a meaningful exception, an AI system may simply flag it as irrelevant noise. Human intelligence and experience are then needed again to do all the tasks that cannot be automated and to work around machines. For healthcare workers, this could lead to burnout, higher turnover rates, and increased spending on recruitment and training. In summary, while automation can enhance efficiency in administrative tasks, the removal of meaningful human engagement in direct care can create inefficiencies, generate additional costs from managing unintended consequences, and ultimately undermine the effectiveness of healthcare systems.

Towards a more equitable PM, and new economies of innovation

The authors of this volume articulate a strong commitment to a future of personalised healthcare that is very different from the kind of 'personalisation' outlined here. They propose a PM that "acknowledges and supports both the heterogeneity and solidarity in society, that liberates rather than dominates, and makes room for its patients rather than excluding or disciplining its subjects" (p9). In the final chapter of this book, they discuss what it takes to build such a future. Affordable and accessible healthcare for all is key. It will need to involve integrating patient-centred care, where patients' holistic needs and social contexts are considered. Meaningful patient and public involvement in healthcare decision-making is also important. Perhaps counterintuitively, this could also help cut cost – in the sense that interventions that people do not really want could be saved. At present, some healthcare services are given to people purely based on eligibility, not because these interventions will improve people's quality of life (e.g. Kaufman 2020). A substantive and systematic consideration of people's needs and values – which I have called 'social biomarkers' (Prainsack 2020) – can help to bring down cost in places where it does not hurt patients.

The authors also call for improved data governance, including dynamic consent and collective oversight, to protect privacy and prevent discrimination. Ultimately, the authors argue for a PM that is humane, equitable, and responsive to the diverse needs of all individuals and communities.

For this to be possible, as the authors show, the way we think and enact economies of innovation needs to change: The current biomedical innovation ecosystem, dominated by private companies and governed by intellectual property rights and market mechanisms, needs to give way to more democratic and equitable model. Instead of prioritising commercial interests and market-driven innovation, the authors advocate for an alternative model of innovation governance that includes stronger public sector involvement and a shift towards a mixed economy of pharmaceutical development. This would entail increased support for socially driven pharmaceutical innovation (SPIN), public-sector research, and regulatory frameworks that promote accessibility rather than reinforcing monopolistic control.

This book reminds us that the future of PM will not be determined by technological innovation alone, but by the social and political choices that guide it. By offering a critical and constructive vision of what a more just and solidaristic form of personalisation could look like, the authors invite us to imagine – and to build – a healthcare future that serves all, not just the privileged few.

Notes

1 To address racialised and other inequities, Dolan and colleagues (2024) recently recommended, among other things, that genetics should be 'de-weaponised' by making it less exploitable by white nationalists and far-right movements by reforming research practices that make race appear to be genetic.

2 Mette Nordahl Svendsen and colleagues critique 'selective medicine', which emphasises using predictive technologies to identify and manage risks at the individual level. They argue that this approach creates distinctions between who is considered 'worthy' of medical attention and resources based on measurable risk factors. This can lead to unequal access to care, prioritising those deemed more 'valuable' by data-driven criteria while neglecting others. Svendsen and colleagues advocate for a broader understanding of health that acknowledges social and ethical complexities, ensuring fairness and inclusivity in medical decision-making (Dam et al 2022).

3 In another place we have proposed the creation of a new profession, health information counsellors, for this purpose. See Fiske et al (2019).

AUTHOR CONTRIBUTIONS

Michael Morrison and **Saheli Datta Burton** wrote the main manuscript except the foreword and series editor's preface.

Elisa Lievevrouw was the lead author on Chapter 3 'Infrastructures and Infrastructur-*ing*'.

Elisabetta Biasin was the lead author on Chapter 6 'Health Data Governance in Personalised Medicine'.

1

THE ORIGINS AND MEANING OF PERSONALISED MEDICINE

> It starts with self-diagnosis powered by data (including via wearable devices), which can already monitor a person for a range of vital markers, coupled with artificial intelligence to deliver diagnoses that are proven to be at least as good as that of clinicians […] Treatment itself is also going digital – for example, by changing people's lifestyles with the help of smartphone apps, or by using technologies such as virtual reality to treat, say, chronic pain. Symptom tracking and journaling are powerful tools to help understand daily routines and how they may affect or trigger certain ailments or conditions. Just as effective: apps or devices that remind patients to take their supplements or medicine at the right time and in the right order. Personalisation can go even deeper, for example, by looking at a patient's unique genomic makeup to design specific methods of prevention, diagnosis and treatment.
>
> (Wired.com N.D.)

This is one account of 'personalised medicine' (PM); an idea that promises to change the way medicine is practised, delivered, and experienced. Alternative terms that describe similar territory include 'precision medicine', 'stratified medicine', 'P4' medicine (where the 'P's' stands for 'predictive, preventive, personalised, and participatory'), and systems medicine (Erikainen and Chan 2019; Flores et al 2013; Galasso 2024). For the most part, we will use the term 'personalised medicine' to describe endeavours operating under all of these labels, except where it becomes useful to discuss specific elements particular to one or more of these terms. The transformative promise of personalised (or precision, etc.) medicine is fundamentally linked to new technologies, from genomic databases and wearable trackers to stem cells. Accordingly, the accounts provided in this handbook will focus heavily on technologies of PM. Most commonly when we think of (medical) 'technologies', we

DOI: 10.4324/9781003279556-1

think of physical artefacts like the stethoscope, or complex mechanical devices like an X-ray scanner. However, in this book, as in social studies of technologies more generally, we take a broader definition of 'technology'. Pharmaceuticals, the formal classifications of disease codified in manuals and textbooks, registries of population health data, and even the statistical calculations of public health, all count as (medical) technologies. Contemporary technologies of PM include not only physical tools for sequencing genes or digital sensors for measuring heart rate and blood pressure, but also the networks of data collection, storage, and distribution, and the statistical calculations of genetic epidemiology or big data analytics that make individual measurements meaningful and medically actionable.

Nonetheless, PM is not only a story of technological change or medical innovation, and this is not necessarily the most elegant lens through which to understand and interrogate it as a phenomenon. PM can be thought of as an umbrella term, a brand or marker of identity that can and has been applied to many different technologies, projects, domains of research, and areas of medical practice. PM encompasses different specific aims, practices, impacts, and outcomes in different times and places, crosses public and private sectors, and looks different in various instantiations. In short it is not one thing, but many. Nonetheless, some general trends can be observed including: (i) the use of tailored or adaptive treatment and care pathways (Prainsack 2017a), especially in oncology (Kerr et al 2021); (ii) data driven segmentation and profiling of disease risk, diagnosis, treatments, and prognosis (Horton and Lucassen 2019); (iii) "orphanisation", which entails the use of genetic data, "biomarkers and companion diagnostics alongside novel drugs, [to] fragment disease categories and drug markets, so that they may qualify for orphan drug status" (Gabe and Martin 2023, p177) leading to novel pharmaceuticals being developed for more narrowly defined patient populations; and (iv) the use of living human biological materials to replace, repair, or mimic specific aspects of an individual patient's biology.

The connecting thread that unites these, and other projects of PM, is the aspiration to adapt and adjust the management of health and disease to align with specificities of individual patients or groups of patients. In order to do this, PM requires both greater volumes and types of data on individuals, and also larger, faster, and sometimes more automated systems for comparing those data points that characterise any given person with population level data, in order to give them meaning. In essence, knowing how many individuals belonging to category 'A' (for example possessing a certain genetic variation) have been diagnosed with disease 'B' allows calculation of how likely an individual assigned to category 'A' is to be diagnosed with disease 'B' in future and the likely symptoms and disease progression. The more different data points that can be used to refine the initial characterisation, the more accurate the classification of risk and diagnosis will be (the 'precision' in precision medicine), and the greater likelihood that a doctor can identify and prescribe a course of treatment that will cure, manage, or prevent symptoms (the latter being the 'predictive' in P4 medicine). Ultimately, the 'personal' in personal medicine is less about the 'whole person' as a social or emotional being and more "the quantified 'person' defined in terms of biological and digital data" (Morrison and Kelly 2021, p103).

There is still much to admire in personalisation as a goal: Who, after all, does not want better, easier, cheaper, or more effective healthcare? Who would not want to avoid disease, pain, and suffering? As ever, the devil is in the details. Realising such futures requires considerable work. It requires substantial changes not only in technologies but also in the way healthcare is organised, provided, and experienced. Such changes have social, economic, legal, regulatory, political, as well as scientific and medical consequences. There will be costs as well as benefits, and, as is often the case, these may not be equally distributed across all parts of society. As with all futures, the road ahead is uncertain and complex. This is especially the case for futures that rely on as-yet-unconducted scientific experiments. As the philosopher of science, Hans Jorg Rheinberger has argued, any scientific experiment whose outcome is already known is not really an experiment[1] (1997). Therefore, all scientific futures are subject to some degree of uncertainty, and indeed unknowability. That said, it does not mean the promises of PM are not amenable to critical analysis. Promissory discourses like those associated with PM are necessarily optimistic; difficulties, ambiguities, and uncertainties are usually occluded or marginalised. Critical engagement with such discourses can add context by surfacing implicit assumptions and examining which groups' interests are represented and which are not, who is anticipated to benefit, and who might be ignored or marginalised. That is the task of the following section.

The promise of personalised medicine

The promises and future-orientated claims of PM are much more than mere speculation. They have a specific purpose; to enrol support from disparate groups, and coordinate and motivate actions in the present intended and designed to bring about the desired future(s) (Borup et al 2006; van Lente 1993). In contemporary biomedicine, promise is in large part associated with technologies; hope for better health is thoroughly bound up with aspirations of scientific and technological improvements and advances (Delvecchio-Good 2001). It is worth noting at this juncture that expectations do not exist 'out there', but are crafted and disseminated by specific persons and institutions through particular instantiations: press releases, media briefings and news stories, peer reviewed scientific journal articles and editorials, popular science stories, professional conferences, workshops, government briefing and policy papers, thematic grant calls from national agencies and charitable trusts that fund scientific research, books, podcasts, and many other outlets. Some sets of expectations only apply to a particular technology or project while an overarching and adaptable idea like PM is capable of being applied to different technologies and projects in different places and at different times.

Usually, the details of the roadmap for how to get from 'here' to 'there' are initially broad: investing in an area of research, building a particular type of infrastructure, supporting a programme of technology development or a commercial sector, with a view to adding specificities as progress gets underway. Given that discourses of personalised and precision medicine have been around for some time, many PM strategies and technologies have already been implemented. This handbook cannot be only a discussion of what might be, but also of what is and, indeed, what has been. The examples and cases studied in this handbook will cover PM projects in various stages of development including those which have already been implemented in routine medical care.

Almost all contemporary science and innovation needs support from different groups: academic scientists, companies, state and charitable funding sources, and so on. Technological expectations like those embedded in PM must appeal to the priorities and concerns of these different audiences in order to stimulate coordinated activity across groups and sectors (Tarkkala et al 2019). This requires a degree of interpretive flexibility; that is the broader promise of a narrative like PM must be capable of subtle shifts in framing that appeal to different audiences. For medical professionals there is the promise of faster, more accurate diagnosis, better ability to predict future health problems, and avoid adverse drug reactions (ADRs) by getting the 'right drug to the right patient' reflected especially in the 'precision' aspect of precision medicine (Tutton 2014). For scientists, especially academic scientists, there is the lure of new areas of study, new opportunities for funding, publications, collaborations, and accompanying prestige and career advancement. Universities too need to compete for funding and students, and actively supporting PM initiatives can be a means to enhance or sustain an institution's reputation as a 'cutting edge' research organisation. Moreover, many universities also generate income from out-licensing of patents produced through academic research on novel technological fields conducted by their staff. For the private sector, PM is an area of technological development that opens up new markets for digital healthcare products and services, new opportunities for intellectual property rights, and a chance for entrepreneurs to set up new companies or grow and diversify the offerings of existing firms. For governments and other healthcare payers, investing in and supporting PM is configured as a means to reduce the incidence of disease in populations, avoid ineffective or suboptimal medical care, and reduce ever-growing national healthcare costs.

For all these audiences there is also an accompanying fear that ignoring PM will lead to being 'left behind' and losing prestige and revenue to other companies, scientists or institutions, or falling behind other countries in terms of healthcare provision or as a site for commercial investment. For patients and the public there may also be an appeal to accuracy and avoiding harm of misdiagnosis or ADRs, as well as a general lure of technological progress that underpins the entire narrative (cf. Delvecchio-Good 2001). A successful promissory narrative, then, is one that can integrate such different dimensions of what a 'desirable' future might look like, while remaining at least superficially coherent.

Technological expectations are of course closely linked to hyperbole. Technological hype has been criticised in many quarters for raising unrealistic expectations, which when they inevitably fail to materialise can lead to mistrust or cynicism about the institutions of science and medicine. This is certainly an issue, but evincing more 'realistic' expectations about technological futures, medical or otherwise, is not so simple. Futures are only graspable through methods of projection that are anchored in the present; it is not possible to access a 'real' future devoid of assumptions, calculations, and judgements about what matters and what does not (Brown 2003; Selin and Pereira 2013). That is something we necessarily acknowledge and embrace as part of the mission of this handbook.

Why do we need a critical account of personalised medicine and what does it look like?

This book is a critique of PM, but that does not mean it is an argument *against* PM, much less a rejection of scientific or medical possibility. In keeping with the overall stance of this book, (medical) technologies are not regarded as 'bad', but neither are they an unmitigated good. Nor is it sufficient to repeat the popular view that technologies are morally neutral and that it is only individuals (or sometimes 'societies') that put technologies to good or bad uses (Miller 2021). Designers play an important role in determining the social effects of technology. By 'designers' we mean scientists, engineers, statisticians, physicians, and others working on a technology across (any of the) various stages of its development. Scholars in the field of Science and Technology Studies have long held, and demonstrated by way of case studies, that designers not only make technical decisions about the content of a technology during its development, but that in making these choices they must also anticipate and plan for the social context of the technology's use:

> A large part of the work of innovators is that of 'inscribing' this vision of (or prediction about) the world in the technical content of the new object [...] Thus, like a film script, technical objects define a framework of action together with the actors and the space in which they are supposed to act.
>
> *(Akrich 1992, p208)*

Technology developers are in this sense 'heterogeneous engineers' (Law 1987), integrating and balancing scientific, material, economic, legal, and other concerns in the design process. These decisions are 'value laden' in that they are necessarily normative calculations about what is worth doing and how the technology should look and function, as well as anticipating the roles and capacities of the people with whom the technology is intended to interact. These decisions can have real, if not necessarily intended, consequences when a technology is released into the wider world. For example, in her book *Invisible Women*, Caroline Criado Perez reports that women involved in serious car crashes are 50% more likely than men to incur a serious injury as a result of the crash. One of the reasons for this is that car safety features had, until recently, been designed around an average male Caucasian body standard and were not well adapted to women's, typically smaller, lighter range of body sizes (Criado Perez 2019). This is not to say that car safety technologies like airbags are 'bad', but rather that women were not adequately anticipated or figured as 'users' of car safety features by designers and were thus unable to benefit equally from the technology in its original iteration. The world of artificial intelligence (AI) also provides numerous recent examples. To list just one in detail, an AI tool employed in some US healthcare settings was used to identify patients with high expected medical needs. The tool did this by assigning a risk score on the basis of total healthcare costs accrued in one year. Healthcare costs were taken as a valid proxy for anticipated healthcare needs because higher costs are generally associated with greater health needs. However, while average health costs for both black and white patients were similar, the average black patient had more, and more severe, conditions than the average white patient (Ledford 2019). By using healthcare costs as a proxy for need, the AI systematically underestimated the level of need of black patients. The authors of the study that identified this problem considered the effect as resulting from a combination of increased socio-economic burdens in accessing healthcare and ethnicity effects on doctor–patient interactions in the US healthcare systems, which meant that black patients on average generate lower health costs than white patients with the same illnesses (Obermeyer et al 2019). In this case, the choice of proxy measure was a source of unfairness and discrimination, even though on initial examination it appeared to perform fairly (i.e. there was no disparity in average cost across ethnic groups) and was not necessarily the result of any conscious intent to discriminate.

Once PM, in all its various technologies and projects, is recognised as a social and political endeavour as much as a scientific and technological one, it becomes possible to aspire to a better politics of PM. As noted above, it is not possible to imagine, or indeed to discuss, any future devoid of assumptions, calculations, and judgements about what matters and what does not. It is, therefore, important to make clear our own commitments to what a desirable future might look like, and equally what we consider undesirable. The perspective taken in this handbook is that a 'better' PM involves a medicine that acknowledges and supports both heterogeneity and solidarity in society, liberates rather than dominates, and makes room for its patients rather than excluding or disciplining its subjects. This approach necessarily rejects the outdated conception that technologies develop through some ineluctable internal logic, that their form and function are determined solely by immutable scientific laws, and that our only real choice is to accept their inevitability and learn to live with them. Understanding that technological and social orders mutually inform one another, and that social and political considerations shape technologies as much as technologies shape our forms of life, the societal responsibility for technological development and its consequences becomes clear. It is possible to choose not only between different forms of a technology, but also between different avenues of technological development, including the option not to cultivate certain technologies at all (De Saille and Medvecky 2016). This supports the argument for more democratic governance of innovation, for greater collective input into the design of technologies and the wider systems through which they are produced, made available, used, assessed, maintained, and disposed of.

The analysis in this book will consider both positive and negative aspects of PM as it is currently envisaged and practised. These issues take a range of forms. Some are technical and practical: if vast data collection is required for a particular PM project, it is reasonable to query whether any existing system can accommodate the proposed volume of information, or, if extensive new infrastructure is needed, to ask who will pay for designing, implementing, operating and maintaining it. And if the funds are to come out of existing healthcare budgets, what services are we opting not to pay for in order to fund these new projects? Some are organisational or procedural challenges, a category that includes the necessity to consider the legality and the impact of regulation on technology development and use. Others are societal and moral: instances where particular versions of PM might be technically and economically feasible but where there is significant likelihood of often intangible, but all too real harms to individuals or to particular groups, such as discrimination, bias, exclusion, misdiagnosis, over- or under-treatment, loss of privacy, and so on. Often challenges can occupy more than one category, as for example the issue of distributed liability in algorithm-assisted medical decision-making, which is both a legal and an ethical issue (Bleher and Braun 2022). A further category of challenges to be explored in this book is the conceptual challenges to ideas underpinning PM itself. Part of our task is to unpack what 'personalisation' in contemporary medicine means. PM is not just a vision of technological medicine; most of its iterations and the different technology platforms being developed under the banner of PM emphasise the role of increasing volumes of information and digital technologies in collecting, processing, and analysing this information to produce particular forms of 'personalisation' in healthcare. Unpacking the power and promise of PM means critically examining the ideas of measurement, quantification, classification, calculation, and prediction that underpin this 'data-driven' digital imaginary. For the most part, the scope of our analysis is not intended to show that PM cannot, or should not, work (although some specific cases may show that PM cannot work in certain ways). Instead, they are presented in the spirit of critique that illuminates and clarifies problems in order to address them. The final chapter of this book will consider alternative ways in which PM might be imagined and materialised, if informed by values of solidarity, shared responsibility, and privileging an ethos of care over the logic of consumer choice.

Here it is necessary to add an important caveat in relation to the book's scope. As per the subtitle of this handbook, we are primarily focused on manifestations of PM in the global 'north'. This is an imperfect term, as the dichotomy of global north and south implies a degree of homogeneity between countries assigned to each category. This is far from the case. For both the 'north' and 'south' different countries have different economies, climates, healthcare systems, customs and values, modes of government, and more. They differ in the density, size, and diversity of their populations, and in the historical contexts which inform their present circumstances and in a myriad of other ways too. That said, PM is primarily a programme – or rather, a set of different programmes and initiatives – aimed at reconfiguring healthcare practices and delivery in developed post-industrial economies, where infectious diseases have not, until the recent advent of COVID-19, been a major healthcare concern since the nineteenth century and there is an expectation of high availability of resources and capital to be invested in healthcare innovation. While there are clearly initiatives that engage at least some of the elements of PM described above being implemented in low- and middle-income countries (notable examples would include the China Kadoorie Biobank or the H3Africa population genomics consortia), a detailed survey of how PM is or might be implemented in these diverse contexts is beyond the scope and expertise of this work.

Having established our topic and aims, the remainder of this chapter will review key developments in the emergence of contemporary western medicine leading up to, and including, the emergence of pharmacogenetics and pharmacogenomics (PgX), which heralded the first widespread discussions, and implementation, of PM. The final section will then provide a brief overview of the structure and content of the subsequent chapters in this handbook.

A brief history of (im)personal medicine

A large part of the intrinsic appeal of labels like 'personalised medicine' and 'precision medicine' is the implication that existing healthcare is *impersonal* and *imprecise*. In order to unpack this, it is useful to briefly revisit the history of modern biomedicine. Sickness has, for human beings, both a social and often a moral meaning, and it affects the network of social relations in which individuals are embedded during their everyday life (Lupton 2003; Turner 1995). Being ill affects (usually by reducing) the body's capabilities and an individual's ability to perform social actions, such as work or participation in family activities. Sickness can also affect identity, marking a person out as someone requiring care or as someone who has transgressed to 'bring the disease upon themselves'. The human body and those instances of heightened awareness about the body that mark the experience of illness and disease have been the objects of medical attention for centuries and indeed provide the *raison d'être* for medical practice: "There has never been a time that men and women have not suffered from sickness, and the physicians' specialised social role has developed in response to it" (Rosenberg 1992, pxiii). However, for historical reasons much of what follows foregrounds how medicine's social role evolved in the western, European context.

It would be a mistake to over-emphasise the continuity in this account: medicine, in Europe as elsewhere, has not followed a systematic process of enlightenment, arriving at its present conjunction by a gradual elucidation of the truth while progressively discarding incorrect theories. Rather, medicine has existed in a series of different, discontinuous forms at different times and places, each with its own epistemological regime and related practices. The form of western medicine preceding the eighteenth century has been described as "library medicine" "in which the classical learning of the physician seemed more important than any specific knowledge of illness" (Armstrong 1995, p393). During the eighteenth century this was supplanted by a medicine displaying greater concern with managing and classifying illnesses, especially through the work of English doctor Thomas Sydenham, who promoted the idea of diseases as distinct entities recognisable by common patterns of symptoms (Reiser 1993). This is an important step in the emergence of modern medicine. Prior to the advent of hospital medicine, illnesses were seen as idiosyncratic phenomena, understood in terms of the particular symptoms reported by the patient; thus, a complaint of stomach pain meant that stomach pain was the disease to be treated by the doctor (Armstrong 2006; King 2006). Disease, and often treatment, was seen as unique and specific to that patient. Recognising patterns of disease symptoms, progression, and response to different interventions allows the beginning of disease classification and the comparison of the effectiveness (or otherwise) of treatment courses by looking at the responses of different patients with comparable conditions. Diagnosis could now operate by assigning patients into existing disease categories.

At the end of the eighteenth century and primarily in Paris, a new form of medicine arose, based on the anatomical model of the body and located in the hospital (Armstrong 1995; Foucault 1973). The growth of large urban centres such as London and Paris also prompted the rise of what we would now consider public health as a direct response to the inescapable problems of bodies dwelling in close proximity: infectious disease, sanitation, birth and mortality rates, race, and lifespan. Accompanying the urbanisation and industrialisation of western society, a range of social changes – including state-applied universal age markers for the beginning and end of school attendance, voting age, and qualification for public pensions – brought greater visibility (not least in institutional terms) to the different elements of the life course (Cole 1992). Such techniques of social stratification allowed the development of medical classification systems detailing "lists of illnesses that are more closely associated with the body at certain times during life – diseases of childhood and of the elderly, and the different diseases of men and women in 'midlife'" (Brown and Webster 2004, p4). This, in turn, allowed the structuring of public health provision around these general categories. The idea of a standardised life course provides a basis for models of 'normal' development and 'abnormal' variation, which can be used as the rationale for medical intervention (Vincent 2006). Thus, it was not only diseases that could now be organised into groups and categories, but also patients and indeed the wider population. This intersection is further evidenced by the emergence of new medical specialities such as paediatrics and geriatrics, dedicated to the health – and diseases – of particular subsets of the population stratified and organised by age range and socio-cultural status, as children or the elderly (Mahnke 2000; Morley 2004).

The processes of medical categorisation were amply aided by that other great tool of public health – statistics. Two nineteenth century pioneers of public health, Louis-Rene Villermé and Adolphe Quetelet, had already begun the application of statistical means to study the effects of living conditions on health, primarily assessed through measurement of physical characteristics including height and weight (Tanner 1981). Quetelet is chiefly renowned for adapting the normal distribution curve, which was originally developed to describe errors of astronomical observations, to describe the distribution of such characteristics in a population in terms of deviation from a central, average (normal) set of values (Hacking 2006). Francis Galton introduced further statistical refinements to the analysis of populations, including the concepts of standard deviation, which describes the extent of difference from the average, and the correlation coefficient, which provides a measure of the reliability of inferring a connection between two sets of quantitative data, such as weight and incidence of heart disease. Statistical calculations could thus link population segments classified by age, socio-economic status, or behaviours not only to the incidence of illness, but also to the *risk* of illness and the *potential* of individuals in those categories to pose a threat to health. It is no coincidence that this era saw the rise of accounting, actuarial attempts at rational calculation of risk and the insurance industry (Brown and Webster 2004).

The introduction in the nineteenth century of a range of technologies for physical diagnosis added a further important element. Medical technologies, then as now, afford physicians new capabilities and ways of knowing. However, they do not, in themselves, mandate any particular way of organising medical care, nor do they determine relationships between physicians and patients. They do provide an impetus and a focal point for projects of reorganisation and reordering. First the stethoscope and ophthalmoscope, and later X-rays and laboratory tests, removed the physician's dependence on the patient's account in making diagnostic judgements. Given that the discourse of science, and scientific medicine, relies for much of its authority on the assumption that the knowledge it produces is objective, universal, and acultural, this transition to technologically mediated medicine alleviated much of the prior dependence on patients to provide personal (and thus subjective) accounts of their symptoms and illness. Diagnostic assessment of individual patients was thus able to focus more on what was the same about each patient, not on what was unique. These, and other new technologies, facilitated the replacement of individuals' self-reported symptoms by standardised measurements and categorisations, such as age, height, race, gender, or physical signs of disease, which in turn aligned with the application of standardised categories of diseases.

This reification of broad disease categories also paved the way for mass production of pharmaceuticals targeted at the standardised 'typical patient'. Advances in inorganic chemistry gave rise to the capacity to produce industrial quantities of small molecule compounds, which, if they had medicinal properties, could be sold as pharmaceuticals. Larger existing pharmaceutical companies at the start of the twentieth century were attracted to the idea of scientific standards, in both manufacturing and evidence for treatment efficacy, not least as a way of distinguishing themselves from patent medicines made of secret (undisclosed) ingredients and the general suspicion of charlatanry accompanying many pharmaceutical enterprises at the time. Only they had the resources to comply with the new regulatory requirements to present appropriate experimental human and animal safety data (as required for example by the 1938 Federal Food, Drug, and Cosmetic Act in the US) because they had recruited scientific staff and had a working relationship with academic medical departments, while their competitors did not. Academic and clinical researchers for their part were often happy to turn over, or at least out-licence, the production of new chemical therapies they had discovered to pharmaceutical firms. For example, this is exactly what happened with insulin, one of the first 'wonder drugs' of twentieth century medicine. In 1922 Frederick Banting, together with his colleagues, produced and successfully tested an alcohol-based extract of bovine pancreas on a number of patients with diabetes (Bliss 1983). The discovering researchers took out a patent on their method of production through the University and licensed production of their discovery to a commercial manufacturer, US-based company Eli Lilly. Laboratory researchers faced restrictions on the amount of raw material they could practically obtain and process and would also have faced significant expense in attempting large scale preparation of the new drug (Oudshoorn 1994). By licensing their discoveries to industrial manufacturers, they were able to relieve themselves of this burden and gain financial recompense for their discoveries which often took the form of increased research funds paid through the patent-holding universities. In return, companies such as Eli Lilly gained preferential access to a new scientifically validated drug with a large patient population defined by standardised, established diagnostic criteria – in other words, a ready-made market.

Thus, by the early twentieth century, technologies of measurement and diagnosis, classifications of diseases and patients, accompanying medical specialisations, and the domains of hospital medicine, public health, and a pharmaceutical industry developing scientific medicines for broadly defined patient populations had entered the picture, bringing us closer to something we might recognise as modern biomedicine. This rationalised, standardised, technology-orientated approach to healthcare, accompanied by industrially mass produced and globally distributed pharmaceuticals, has proved enormously successful and has been institutionalised, to varying degrees, at a global level. However, this rise was not without its critics, who suggested that western biomedicine also produced an 'impersonalised medicine', where the focus on established diagnostic categories and set, approved treatment protocols allowed only limited scope for relations of interpersonal care between doctors and their patients (Tutton 2014). The stage was set for the first wave of genetic technologies to usher in a move towards greater stratification of large patient populations, with accompanying selection of treatment options that gave rise to the modern idea of PM.

Pharmacogenetics, pharmacogenomics, and the beginnings of personalised medicine

The western-dominated pharmaceutical industry that emerged after the Second World War was based, as discussed above, on small molecule chemical drugs tested and marketed primarily in broadly defined diagnostic categories. These small-molecule drugs were mass produced in centralised, industrial manufacturing sites and fed into increasingly global supply chains, meaning that all patients assigned to a particular disease category could expect to receive a medicine that was for all practical purposes 'the same' regardless of where they lived or which physician or hospital they visited; the very antithesis of PM. While these medicines demonstrated sufficient efficacy to secure market approval by national medicines regulators such as the US Food and Drug Administration, it was also recognised that they produced undesirable side effects in many recipients. Most approved medicines come with a list, sometimes an extensive list, of possible side effects, the anticipated severity of each possible adverse effect, and its frequency in the population of patients taking that drug. The more serious of these unwanted effects are known as ADRs and can lead to serious medical complications, and even fatalities. In this sense most approved medicines 'work' (that is they adequately remove, alleviate, or modulate the symptoms of the condition they are applied to treat) but they do not work equally well for everyone in a given patient population. Judging whether the benefits outweigh the harms is part of the job, and the justification, for medicines regulators, but it is also an illustration of the tension between the general (the collective of patients considered to have a given disease) and the particular (each individual patient who does or does not respond well to the drug) that will be a recurring feature of discussions on PM.

The idea that different responses to a given drug might be due to genetic differences between patients is not a new one. The use of the term 'pharmacogenetics' to describe the effect of genetics on drug metabolism was reported as early as 1959, only six years after Watson and Crick first reported the molecular structure of DNA itself (Hedgecoe 2004). Techniques for sequencing and 'reading' DNA started to become available in the 1970s, but they were slow, labour intensive, and could only handle short sequences. The completion of the Human Genome Project in 2003 and the advent of genomics, including ever faster genetic sequencing techniques, gave new impetus to the search for links between genetics and patients' responses to drugs, as well as giving rise to a related endeavour pharmacogenomics. Both, somewhat confusingly, have been abbreviated to 'PGx' (Hedgecoe 2003). Where pharmacogenetics aims to identify specific variants of a given gene that affect whether a patient responds well or poorly to a given drug (either not benefiting or having an ADR), pharmacogenomics looks at the interactions between the whole genome and a given small molecule compound (Lindpaintner 2004). The two fields are closely intertwined, making use of the same underlying technological platforms.

Arguably, pharmacogenomics proved to be the more successful endeavour: testing potential new drug candidate molecules against multiple genes and gene variants allowed drug developers to stratify common complex diseases into subtypes associated with different gene variants. New drugs that affected these genetic subtypes, often by interacting with a protein or a cell surface receptor produced by the targeted gene variant, could then be developed for particular subsets of patients with a condition. This form of molecular 'matching' between genetic variant and drug mechanism is one of the approaches that are considered personalised or tailored medicine. Pharmacogenomic 'targeting' was particularly successful in the field of oncology, which is unsurprising given the dominant understanding of cancer as a genetic disease and the fact that even small extensions in lifespan or quality of life can make a difference – and command strong reimbursement – for cancer care. Imatinib mesylate (marketed in the United States as Gleevec and as Glivec outside the United States) and Trastuzumab (trade name Herceptin) are both examples of commercially successful cancer therapies that target a specific molecular signature in a subset of patients with leukaemia and breast cancer, respectively. Chronic myeloid leukaemia (CML), a subcategory of leukaemia, can be diagnosed by the presence of a chromosomal abnormality known as the 'Philadelphia chromosome', which produces a mutant and overactive protein (Charatan 2001). This abnormal protein is responsible for triggering the excessive cell proliferation characteristic of cancer and is also the target of Imatinib. Trastuzumab is a monoclonal antibody that attacks breast cancer tumours expressing high levels of human epidermal growth factor receptor 2 (HER2). Trastuzumab also comes with its own associated genetic test to identify HER2-positive breast cancer patients, showing how pharmacogenetic testing and pharmacogenomics intertwine.

Other pharmacogenetic tests were also developed, targeting particular genes associated with drug metabolism in humans such as those in the Cytochrome P450 family. The idea is that fast or slow metabolism of drugs affected by this family of genes, which includes common medications for heart disease and antidepressants, could result in patients getting the drug out of their system before it has time to induce a therapeutic effect or conversely not breaking it down fast enough causing a build up to dangerous, ADR-inducing levels. This allows patients to be stratified into 'rapid', 'normal', or 'slow' metabolisers and given adjusted dosages or assigned to a different medicine entirely. Another example of an established pharmacogenetic test is that for the thiopurine methyltransferase (TPMT) gene. Thiopurines are a class of drugs used to treat leukaemia. Despite general success, a small number of patients have been found to suffer dangerous, even fatal toxicity as a result of thiopurine drug treatment. The enzyme thiopurine methyltransferase (coded for by the TPMT gene) is responsible for metabolising the thiopurine drugs in the body (van Aken 2003). A pharmacogenetic test is able to identify different variants (alleles) of the TPMT gene, some of which are associated with slow metabolism and resulting in dangerous ADRs.

As this brief overview illustrates, the cases of pharmacogenetics and pharmacogenomics display many of the key aspirations and techniques of PM: stratification of patient populations based on biological (here genetic) data, novel testing regimes, existing medical treatment regimens (such as dosage of choice of drug) adjusted to particular patient subgroups on the basis of this information, and in some cases the development of novel therapeutics targeting specific molecular mechanisms associated with stratified disease subtypes. However, many of the limitations of PM projects are also evident. Only a portion of variation in drug response between patients can be reliably attributed to specific genetic differences. For example, with TPMT testing, a minority of total adverse reactions suffered by patients taking thiopurines are actually due to genetic variants of the TPMT gene; the rest are due to other factors such as interactions with other medicines and variants in other genes (van Aken 2003). Moreover, as this last example also shows, a relatively small proportion of genetic variation in response can be linked solely, or even mainly, to variations in a single gene. The reliability of pharmacogenetic tests depends on the quality and representativeness of the pool of genetic data used to make connections between genes and responses to drugs, meaning that the accuracy and usefulness of tests is often lower in non-Caucasian populations. The economic case for pharmacogenetic tests has also been patchy; Verbelen et al (2017) found that of the 137 associations between genetic variants and drugs that have so far been incorporated into the prescribing advice labels issued with FDA-approved pharmaceuticals, only some had a published cost–benefit analysis while for many no such data was available. In other cases, several analyses were available for the same test and drug combination but the conclusions they reached were not in agreement. So, while pharmacogenetics had some modest successes, it did not herald a revolutionary change in medicine, where each new drug would come with its own bespoke genetic test.

The pharmacogenomic approach of stratifying patient population into subgroups defined by genetic or other biological markers has had a greater lasting impact, as will be discussed in Chapter 5, and was more commercially successful. However, while the clinical benefit of targeted medicines can indeed be substantial for patients in the affected subgroup, the outcomes can be less positive for those who have other forms of the disease, and indeed for the clinicians who are treating them. Trastuzumab has little benefit for breast cancer patients who do *not* have high levels of HER2, but their condition is no less serious despite not gaining any new therapies. In this way PM can create new currents of marginalisation and neglect for those patients who do not have the 'right' genetic variant to receive an improved treatment regime or product (Dickenson 2013). Moreover, once a targeted medicine receives marketing approval, there is relatively little incentive for firms to produce robust evidence of its utility (or not) in other patient populations. Trastuzumab was approved for women with HER2 positive breast cancers in 1998 but accumulating enough evidence that women with HER2 negative cancers did not receive any significant benefit took a further 20 years of work (Kimmelman and

Tannock 2018). Ultimately, the rise of pharmacogenetics and pharmacogenomics did much to popularise the idea of PM and set in place many of the broad trends that still characterise contemporary developments in the field, even as PGx has somewhat faded from view. These subsequent developments form the substantive topic for the remaining chapters in this handbook.

Evidence-based medicine and patient-centred healthcare

Before summarising the book's subsequent contents, it is useful to clarify two other developments in healthcare that are distinct from PM, but which nonetheless interact with it in different ways: evidence-based medicine (EBM) and patient-centred healthcare. EBM is a movement that initially emerged from Canada in the early 1990s, and which has at its heart the aim of placing experimental clinical evidence as the primary basis for medical decision-making. While few doctors would claim their practice was not evidence driven, EBM imposes a specific hierarchy of evidence types, with double-blinded randomised placebo controlled clinical trials as the highest standard of evidence and experience-based judgement making much lower down the scale (Goldenberg 2006). EBM is important to discussions of PM firstly because of its success. As Mykhalovskiy and Weir (2004, p1059) explain:

> EBM has grown into one of the most important and successful initiatives to recompose contemporary biomedical reasoning and practice [, it] has been met with remarkable enthusiasm on the part of the elites in academic medicine [and] has been formally incorporated into editorial policies, has spawned new journals and approaches to reporting biomedical research, and is now routinely taught throughout medical schools in North America, the UK and parts of Western Europe.

Moreover, this success means that EBM informs the medical and scientific environment from which most PM endeavours emerge and provides criteria against which their success will be measured by medical professionals, healthcare policy makers, regulators, and others. On the one hand, EBM provides for new waves of medical standardisation and depersonalisation, which seem to stand in contrast to the aims of PM, but on the other hand, as subsequent chapters of this book will illustrate, much PM is not a rejection of the classifying, ordering mode of twentieth century medicine, but an intensification of it, one that actively requires and produces new standards and classifications to underpin the ever greater stratification of patient populations and diseases. As such EBM can both support and challenge particular projects of PM in different ways, as later chapters of this book will illustrate and discuss.

Patient-centred healthcare is a movement that aims to give patients greater say in decision-making about their care, and in defining and assessing what counts as 'quality' in healthcare. This mirrors, and in some degree is a response to, a more activist role of patient groups and charities, whose 'traditional' roles of providing support and information to patients themselves is increasingly accompanied by mobilisation of collective 'experiential knowledge' in support of their particular claims, raising funds to support scientific and medical research and lobbying for patient rights in pursuit of better care and therapies (Moreira 2015; Rabeharisoa et al 2014). However, the rhetoric of 'participation' is also used to valorise efforts to encourage, or even mandate, patients and members of the public taking greater direct responsibility for managing their own health (Oborn and Barrett 2016; Prainsack 2014). This can include collecting, recording, and making available data about their biological characteristics and medical history to academic and commercial researchers, engaging with and purchasing commercial services like direct-to-consumer genetic tests, wearable sensors and self-tracking apps, and other tools for self-management. Some of these types of activities are alluded to by the 'participatory' in P4 medicine. However, as will be discussed further in Chapter 4, this 'responsibilisation' of citizens and patients can also be an excuse for governments to cut services and reduce spending on health and social infrastructure, dismissing those who are not able, for reasons of poor health, poverty, or environmental restrictions, to be 'active participants' in their own care as 'unwilling' or 'irresponsible' and undeserving of support (Prainsack 2014).

Structure of this book

The subsequent chapters of this book are organised in the following way: Chapters 2–6 will each focus on a specific theme relating to PM, while Chapter 7 ties together insights from across the book to address the question 'what does a better PM look like?' We have chosen not to dedicate individual chapters to particular technologies (such as genomics) or to specific case studies (such as the All of US Precision Medicine Initiative) but to orientate each chapter around a particular aspect of PM: its conceptual underpinnings, infrastructures, publics, and so on. The roster of PM projects and technologies is constantly changing and evolving. Trying to cover every example, even limited to the 'global north', would be both impossible and very soon out of date. Equally, dealing only with a small subset of 'exemplar' case studies in detail would give only a partial, and biased account of what PM involves and means. Instead, the thematic approach provides a series of critical lenses through which to understand and interrogate PM that can be applied across a range of projects, technologies, and instantiations beyond those explicitly discussed in this work.

Chapter 2 delves deeper into the 'data driven' nature of much contemporary PM. Continuing the idea, outlined in this chapter, that PM is less a genuine rupture with the medicine of the twentieth century and more an intensification and expansion of it, the chapter begins with a focus on the role of measurement and quantification. These basic processes inform the creation of categories of diseases and persons and the calculation of risk that underpins modern medicine, personalised, or otherwise. Identifying the social authority of data, especially quantified data, in its claims to be scientific and objective, we consider what these terms actually entail and present an argument that while data clearly constitute a representation of real phenomena and make them legible and comprehensible, they are nonetheless inseparable from issues of judgement and value. This is not intended to denigrate scientific medicine but to introduce a note of epistemic humility, and to deflate grandiose claims that everything could be rendered knowable and calculable if only sufficiently large volumes of data are available. Having established what data can and cannot do, the chapter then turns to issues of diagnosis and risk calculation, drawing on historical as well as more contemporary examples to show how the use of data to organise populations into categories, of health and disease, and of probabilistic risk of illness, is always a process with consequences. It does not simply capture a material reality 'out there' but actively constructs categories that come to have shared social meanings and consequences for personal and group identity (e.g. as patients), for the professional and institutional organisation of healthcare, and, through the administrative bureaucracies of nation states, for resource allocation, the design of public health measures and more. The final section of Chapter 2 considers the increasing automation of data collection and processing, especially with AI. Building on the understandings of data, categorisation, and calculation set out in the earlier sections of this chapter, this section then considers how the algorithmic processing of data exemplifies both the promise and the perils of PM.

Chapter 3 turns to the means by which the data on which PM depends is stored, aggregated, circulated, and made available for use – the infrastructures of PM. Infrastructure is all around us, most obviously in the physical infrastructure of roads, water pipes, mobile phone masts, traffic lights, signs, mailboxes, bus stations, ferry terminals, and many other familiar features of the modern landscape. However, infrastructure also extends to the conceptual, to the standards and classifications that make things 'the same' across time and space, or which, especially for digital technologies, facilitate interoperability across systems (such as between mobile phones on different networks or digital devices with different operating systems). Infrastructure concerns both the systems that organise and connect human societies and the rules for operating and maintaining those systems. A great deal of PM leverages the 'installed base' (Bowker and Star 1999) of the existing infrastructure of medicine established during the nineteenth and twentieth centuries from diagnostic categories to medical records and healthcare facilities. The promise of PM also requires and motivates a range of new infrastructure building projects, and this work of *infrastructuring* – or making infrastructure – is the main focus of Chapter 3. Using two examples of large-scale, state-supported projects of infrastructuring, the All of US Precision Medicine Initiative in the United States and the European Union's Virtual Human Twin Initiative, this chapter reveals that infrastructures, like measurements and categories (which are after all a form of infrastructure), are value-laden endeavours. Infrastructure building has politics and, importantly for the users, data subjects, and patients whose care is mediated by infrastructures of PM, it has consequences. Through the All of US case study we examine efforts to embed ideas of socioeconomic, ethnic, and gender-based fairness in a national PM project and how the need for new infrastructure to be built on existing infrastructure risks perpetuating and entrenching unequal access to the benefits of personalisation. The second case study, the Virtual Human Twin Initiative also has a unifying political aim, in this case to draw together existing efforts to create digital 'models' of patients (the titular 'digital twins') to create a unified digital twin infrastructure capable of modelling 'European' patient populations and predicting their responses to different treatment regimes. The aspiration in this second case study is explicitly linked to the aim of generating alternative forms of evidence to support the launch of personalised care programmes and drugs. As we outlined above, PM projects are animated by promise, and promises typically begin life as somewhat vague, abstract, and high-level visions of what a better future could look like. It is only as PM projects move from vision to action that the rhetoric of promise is moulded through the reality of practice and starts to take shape as real structures, technical systems, and rules. It is through infrastructuring work that PM projects take shape and where their real-world impacts are determined, making infrastructuring an important site to study the politics of PM.

As part of their politics, infrastructures of PM encode particular visions of the populations they are intended to serve (or surveil), and these 'persons' envisaged by PM are also, appropriately, the focus of the next chapter. Chapter 4 explores some of the different ways in which visions of PM present their users – their 'publics' – as research subjects, as consumers, and as citizens, and unpacks the scripts (Akrich 1992) associated with these different configurations. Taking different visions in turn, the chapter examines how commercial PM services, such as direct-to-consumer genetic tests, configure their users as 'consumers', who take personal responsibility for their health and act on this by purchasing products and services to preserve or enhance their health. These are typically informational goods, presented as a way to empower individuals to make healthier choices. In discourses of public health, governments envisage the public as 'citizens' with both rights (for example the right to adequate healthcare) but also, again, responsibilities, which can be discharged by contributing data to medical research and allowing data from medical care to be aggregated and repurposed as national biomedical big data resources. Echoing Chapter 2, this chapter also argues that participants in PM can come to be viewed as research subjects, constituted first and foremost through the lens of biological data, and classified as either being eligible or ineligible for experimental PM treatment regimens. In their study of cancer care, Dam et al (2022) describe this as making 'precision patients', that is, in practice personalisation can become less about adapting care to each patient and more about selecting which patients have the right biomarkers to benefit from inclusion in PM. Chapter 4 also explores different forms of resistance to PM discourses and practices, from those who object to the transfer and secondary use of their data, to 'biohackers' who embrace the message of individual responsibility for health to the extent that their attempts at self-optimisation frequently exceed the dictates of medical authority. The final section of the chapter turns to the way 'publics' for PM are engaged in practice and how public engagement on issues in science and medicine can be either a genuine attempt at direct democracy or an attempt to manufacture consent for the status quo while side-lining dissent, depending on how these activities are conceived and conducted.

Chapter 5 is something of an exception to the overall pattern, in that it deals with personalised treatments, as distinct from the data-driven stratification, classification, and prediction that characterise the greater part of most PM endeavours covered in this book. Here the focus is on a specific set of technologies, the use of human cells, tissues, and genetic modification as medicinal interventions, a field often collectively described as 'regenerative medicine'. This is a narrower chapter remit than, for example 'infrastructures' or 'publics' but it allows for a historical analysis of this (broad and often contested) field over time, from the early years of tissue engineering and gene therapy research through to contemporary innovations such as gene editing, 3D printing of biological materials, and stem cells. The chapter explores how 'personalisation' of cell and gene therapies has variously been configured, both in terms of immune matching between tissue donor and recipient, and by pharmacogenomic stratification of patient populations for targeted therapeutics. The historical approach allows us to draw out some recurring patterns, such as the interplay between standardisation and personalisation in making targeted therapies, and the hidden work needed to make novel 'disruptive' treatments workable in practice. The chapter also reports on social science work examining how stratification operates as a strategy in negotiating patient access to treatment, something that is increasingly prominent with very high-cost therapies such as cell- and gene-based medicines. Lastly, Chapter 5 introduces the idea that different approaches to personalisation of treatment give greater weight to consumer choice or to public benefit and have different implications for equity of access to medicines, a theme that will be returned to in Chapter 7.

Regulation of PM is the theme of Chapter 6. Given that PM is driven by and dependent on data, the chapter concentrates on the regulatory frameworks that govern data flows, especially healthcare data which is essential for PM research and practice. As discussed in Chapters 2 and 3, PM depends on aggregation of health-related data from whole populations, which is often achieved through large infrastructure building projects. However, a great deal of the information that feeds into PM projects is considered personal data, that is, data relating to a natural (i.e. a living, human) person and is therefore subject to legal rules such as privacy and data protection. Chapter 6 presents the core legal concepts of privacy, data protection, and cybersecurity, explaining their scope and briefly reviewing the ways they are understood in legal systems such as the United States and the European Union. The chapter then considers the nature of health-related data – assessing when it does, and does not, count as personal data and outlining when the data used in PM does and does not fall under various protections. Having established its subject,

Chapter 6 then presents three case studies of data use in PM, each illustrating a different challenge for its regulation. The case of Care.data in the UK illustrates the challenges of ensuring legitimate reuse of health data, while the example of Google DeepMind's collaboration with the Royal Free Hospital considers issues of consent to be a data subject and what is required for the legitimate sharing of personal health data across institutions. In both cases the adequacy of regulation and oversight is clearly connected with issues of meaningful consent and public trust in healthcare institutions engaged in PM projects. The third case study turns to the issue of synthetic data, that is, of health data records generated by AI and used to replace or supplement PM data sets. Synthetic data can, it is hoped, help to create large enough training data sets for PM algorithms when the existing 'real' dataset is too small (for example with rare disease patients) or poor quality (such as with historically marginalised populations). However, as Chapter 6 examines, synthetic data treads a fine line between being too close a mirror of real patients, risking privacy concerns, or not close enough, raising accuracy concerns. Taken together these case studies and the preceding part of the chapter present an overview of current regulation and governance of health data in the context of the transformations ushered in by PM.

The book's final chapter, Chapter 7, turns to the possible futures of PM. The core of our argument throughout this book is that the greatest strength of PM is also the source of its most fundamental limitations. The power of large-scale, data-driven, digital, algorithmic medicine lies in what it can make visible: the oblique correlations and patterns of behaviour, traits, and environment that shape whether, when, and how we become ill, and that can inform our efforts to successfully treat and even prevent disease. There is enormous potential to alleviate human suffering. However, enabling calculations at the scale on which PM depends for its power requires quantification, datafication and automation. These processes as discussed in Chapter 2, involve stripping out messy and contingent elements of the complex phenomena being counted, paring them back to the simpler, more readily communicable numeric (and increasingly digital) format. And yet, phenomena are meaningful to individuals precisely because of, (and through) being embedded in networks of (messy, local, contingent) social relations (Sayer 2011). To put it another way, a lot of what matters to us as persons is our attachments to *specific* things, others, places, ideas, and so on. These relations are not readily quantifiable or scalable and so by excluding them, PM ironically risks also being a site of further *depersonalisation*. This problem is not unique to PM; depersonalisation, in the form of severing or ignoring of social embeddedness, is the inherent violence of scale and haunts all 'scalable' solutions to social problems (Tsing 2012) but is especially acute given the globalising aspirations of PM. Chapter 7 explores several avenues for mitigating this harm, and, in keeping with the constructively critical ethos of this book, envisages what a better PM might look like. Solidarity (Prainsack 2017b) is emphasised as a key concept for filling out the notion of 'the person' in PM. Solidarity in patient-centred care emphasises a holistic approach that recognises each individual patient as being embedded in sets of social relations and that takes account of their particular circumstances and what matters to them beyond the notions of responsible consumers, citizens, or data subjects described in Chapter 4. Alternative innovation models, such as social pharmaceutical innovation (SPIN), are considered as a means to make PMs more affordable and increase patient access to the increasingly expensive therapies presented in Chapter 5. Returning to another theme of Chapter 4, the notion of Responsible Innovation underscores the need for public dialogue about PM projects and infrastructures to encompass the political, economic, and indeed environmental dimensions of PM. Engagement beyond narrow 'ethical' issues of a specific piece of research or infrastructure-building project is needed to allow for meaningful, rather than tokenistic debate, and ultimately for democratic oversight of PM. Lastly, solidarity, this time in relation to data governance, again foregrounds human interconnectedness by recognising the potential for collective harms, interests, and benefits in aggregated personal data, and tries to make room for the regulatory legitimacy of these shared interests in the face of the hegemonic legal model of autonomous, atomised data subjects described in Chapter 6.

PM is as vast as it is varied. There are a great diversity and number of research projects, infrastructure-building endeavours, products, services, healthcare initiatives, public health programmes, and other phenomena in many different locations globally that fall under the scope of personalised, precision, P4, or stratified medicine and similar terms. The prospect of having any impact at all upon such a leviathan, much less nudging it towards progressive ends, can seem daunting in the extreme. It would be naive to imagine that a book could effect such change. However, people – or 'persons' – are not only the subjects of PM endeavours, they are also its architects. It is our hope that by foregrounding the issues raised by PM and providing a lens to help critically interrogate any given PM endeavour, this work can provide a resource for anyone working on or with PM – and especially those charged with addressing its 'ethical, legal, and social issues'. Big changes, after all, are just the aggregated outcomes of many people trying to make things a little better at the small scale, the local, and indeed, the personal level.

Note

1 For example, the 'experiments' conducted by undergraduate life sciences students are not intended to produce any new knowledge but to train students in laboratory techniques by getting them to perform established procedures that were once experimental.

2

THE PERILS AND PROMISE OF DATA-DRIVEN MEDICINE

In the previous chapter, personalised medicine was described as 'data-driven'. By this, we mean that most personalised medicine endeavours extend and intensify modern medicine's programme of measuring, classifying, and stratifying bodies, diseases, people, and populations, by expanding the scope and scale of information employed. For example, in pharmacogenetics we saw how additional information about variants of a limited number specific genes such as those in the Cytochrome P450 family could be used to classify patients into 'fast', 'slow', or 'average' metabolisers of certain pharmaceutical medications. This degree of personalisation or stratification of patients and matching with an appropriate drug dosage is, as Adam Hedgecoe has noted "more a case of buying a small, medium or large T-shirt from the Gap than being fitted for a Saville row suit" (2004, p5). In other words, a limited amount of additional information, in the form of detection and classification of variants of a particular gene, was used to effect a limited, and somewhat crude, stratification of (some) patients and treatment (dosage) pathways. However, the personalised medicine projects that followed on from and superseded pharmacogenetics and pharmacogenomics, draw on new technologies that promise greater volumes of ever more precise data with which to categorise and classify patients. Advances in genetic sequencing technology promise comparative analysis not only of variants of one or two genes, but also of whole patient genomes, and indeed even of the products of genomes through proteomics (all the proteins produced by a cell), metagenomics (all the epigenetic modifications of a genome), transcriptomics (all the RNA transcripts produced in a cell), metabolomics (all the molecules produced by the metabolic action of a cell or tissue), lipidomics (a subset of the metabolome focusing on the fats, fatty acids, waxes, and related molecules produced by a cell or tissue), and more (Higdon et al 2013).

DOI: 10.4324/9781003279556-2

Digitisation of existing health records (including basic social and physical measures of height, weight, gender, ethnicity, age, and potentially lifestyle and mental health data as well) and digital capture of current and ongoing medical encounters (visits to a primary care physician, hospital appointments, and the results of all tests, scans, reported symptoms, diagnoses, medications prescribed, and treatment outcomes) make a wealth of health information searchable and shareable, able to be combined into databases covering large populations and time periods. Much of this work is enabled by the routine collection and storage of large amounts of patient data in electronic databases of administrative and clinical data (Cook and Collins 2015) and by established 'biobanks' of human tissue and extracted genetic and other biological data linked to medical information about the donors. Expectations for digital personalised medicine also involve widespread accessibility of electronic medical records and the development of tools for incorporating less structured data sources such as text-mining tools for documents, websites, or social media feeds (Ohno-Machado 2013) and the linking of "medical, environmental, financial, geographic, and social media information" (Khoury and Ioannidis 2014, p1054). This data, which can also be integrated with genetic, proteomic, and similar data, can be mined for patterns, and correlations suggestive of new diagnostic categories, new predictions of risk and prognostic outcomes, and new ways of stratifying patient populations and diseases. All this can be augmented by wearable sensors that can measure and record biophysical functions such as blood pressure, heart rate, body temperature, and exercise in real time, and often also transmit these data electronically to large databases for amalgamation, curation, and assessment.

Importantly, no amount of information about a person, however precise and accurate, is medically useful unless it can be linked with associated information derived from a wider population. The importance of statistical correlation as a way of giving meaning to data is evident in, for example, genome-wide association studies (GWAS). GWAS collect information on the frequency of different genetic variants within as large a population as possible and look for correlations between variants and disease outcomes. The 'meaning' of a given gene variant is determined by whether any detected pattern of association between people in the population with that gene variant and a given disease outcome (e.g. a diagnosis) is deemed statistically significant. The same approach, in principle, can be expanded to many points of comparison, to locate any given person – or rather the data points derived from a person – in a web of correlations with corresponding population level data. Here we can see the extension and application of the statistical logics that underpin public health and epidemiology, and the influences of the evidence-based medicine movement, in shaping the vision of data-driven personalised medicine. Implementing this type of approach requires large infrastructures of data collection, storage, and annotation to allow such comparisons to be made. These infrastructures will be discussed in more detail in Chapter 3. The calculative and predictive logics underpinning this type of correlation also underpin the drive to collect and process ever more data about persons, their activities, their diseases, responses to treatment, and so on, and to scale this data collection up to ever-larger populations and collections.

This is exemplified in the rise of 'big data' in healthcare. Defined by its volume (consisting of enormous quantities of data), velocity (often created in real-time), variety (being structured, semi-structured and unstructured), veracity (the data can be messy, noisy and contain uncertainty and error), value (many insights can be extracted and the data repurposed), and variability (data whose meaning can be constantly shifting in relation to the context in which they are generated) (Kitchin and McArdle 2016), big data is also another promissory vision, at once "a science, a business, and—importantly—[...] a mythology" (Crawford et al 2014, p1664). It informs and bleeds into discourses and expectations for personalised or precision medicine. Big data, it is hoped will make personalised medicine more precise, more accurate and more beneficial. Part of the promise of this element of precision is increased *control* through a combination of greater volumes of data and instruments of measurement that are more sensitive and access ever further 'inside' their objects of study. As Kuch et al note: "Across numerous domains, the production of new data in 'precision' fields are accompanied by, or in some cases depend upon, the use of sensors which are claimed to increase the certainty of knowledge and decision-making" (Kuch et al 2020, p528). Indeed, some big data advocates argue that sufficiently large quantities of data alleviate the need for scientific or medical theorisation, that algorithmic analyses of sufficiently vast data sets can give us an unmediated window into reality; the promise of perfect knowledge and perfect precision.

It is an enticing prospect. And of course, it is as illusory as it is alluring. The lure of complete control, a totality of knowledge, and predictability is, as Crawford and colleagues (2014) claim, a modern mythology, enticing, but untenable and impossible. In order to explain why this is so, and why, despite this, the idea seems to hold such appeal, even to intuitively make sense, and to exert such a powerful hold over the imaginations of physicians, policymakers, scientists, and entrepreneurs, it is necessary to examine the very foundations of science and modern medicine, indeed of much of what we consider knowledge at all.

Measurement and quantification: what is counted and who counts?

'Precision' derives from the Latin *praecisio* meaning to cut off or divide, actions that transform a whole into discrete units (Vincent 2022). 'Precision' in precision medicine is read in the sense of the ability to reliably discriminate between one state or entity and another, which in turn can be realised as the number and detail of measurements whose increase is seen as improving the chances of a correct or true mirroring of the phenomenon, state, or entity being captured. Measurement, then, is at the heart of personalised, or precision, medicine. Measurements are not necessarily quantified but many are. 'Quantification' here refers to the basic act of counting and also to the more involved process of converting information into numerical form. As argued in the previous chapter, personalised medicine may be 'new' in terms of new technologies, new practices, and new markets and business opportunities, but it is not a genuine conceptual rupture with the medicine of the nineteenth and twentieth centuries. Measuring and counting bodies, symptoms, people, and outcomes is what made diseases legible as discrete phenomenon. It was the development of standardised measures, technologies, and techniques for knowing bodies that enabled the construction of shared classifications of diseases to which patients could be ascribed, and it is contemporary techniques of measuring, quantifying, and calculating through data mining, wearable sensors, genomic sequencing, and other technologies discussed above that enable the reshaping and fragmenting of these categories in personalised medicine.

The power of measurement, especially when quantified as a numerical figure or reading, lies in its objectivity, its claim to capture aspects of the world as they really are. This is the root of its appeal and of many of its difficulties. As Loraine Daston and Peter Galison (2010) have demonstrated, through painstaking historical analysis, the modern idea of 'objectivity' is a concept with a history. It has not always had the meaning(s) we currently import to it, and it contains within its present form an uneasy fusion of different historical notions of objectivity. 'Current usage' as Daston explains

> allows us to apply the word as an approximate synonym for the empirical (or, more narrowly the factual); for the scientific, in the sense of public, empirically reliable knowledge; for impartiality-unto-self-effacement and cold blooded restraint of the emotions; for the rational, in the sense of compelling assent from all rational minds [...], and for the 'really real', that is to say objects in themselves independent of all minds.
>
> *(Daston 1992, p597–598)*

It is necessary to briefly unpack some of these dimensions to understand how the different strands of 'objectivity' form a compelling but problematic whole.

Objectivity refers to both aspects of knowledge claims about the world and to a form of practice; it is something that is *done* rather than an innate property of things or persons. Scientific research is often said to be objective, but this is by way of a description of *how the* research is conducted which then imputes a certain status to the results. Scientific research makes claims about the world. Claims about phenomena that exist independently of the mind that perceives them are considered to be ontologically objective. However, what we often get wrong is that this does not mean such claims are inherently true. Quite the reverse: if something being studied exists independently of what we think or believe about it, then our claims about it are capable of being wrong (Sayer 2011). In fact, it is *only* if entities exist independently of us that we can be mistaken about them; if a phenomenon existed only in our thoughts then whatever we thought about it would always be correct.

All of us experience the world and get a sense of the properties of things. If we lift something, we have a sense of its weight. If we walk from one location to another, we have a sense of the distance between these two places. If we say an object is 'heavy' or a journey is 'not too long', these are claims about things that exist separately from us, that is they are ontologically objective, but these understandings are internal to us as embodied, conscious subjects. They are thus epistemologically subjective: about real things but difficult to share and make public. How well this information, derived from our experience of things in the world, is interpreted by another person depends on them either experiencing the word in a sufficiently comparable manner to us ('yes, I also find this object to be heavy') or knowing our physical tolerances and capacities (to say nothing of our habitual modes of speech) sufficiently well for them to accurately interpret our reported experiences (knowing for example how fast I walk, whether or not I am used to walking long distances, and whether I tend to exaggerate or downplay the difficulty of tasks). Our personal experiences of the properties of the world around us are not, for the most part, imagined or mistaken, that is they are not ontologically subjective, but something else is needed to communicate them with other people in a way that builds a shared picture of the world. There are many ways in which humans have developed to overcome this internal/external barrier, to share collective experience and understanding including, but hardly limited to language, the written word, drawings and depiction, numbers, and measurement. Even the most basic measurements from far antiquity, notches on a bone to record animal hunts or markings on a wooden pole marking the seasonal height of a river, act as a medium for producing collective knowledge, for moving information from the domain of memory and experience into a more durable, sharable form. This is the "public, empirically reliable knowledge" that Daston recognises as scientific. It is testable, produced by interacting with the world, supported by evidence accessible to more than one mind, and most importantly communicable. Measurement, in all its forms from the most basic to the most sophisticated, is a means of making information about the world epistemologically objective (communal, usually through a shared set of referents and practices) and ontologically objective (about things that exist independently of what we believe about them). This is a huge advantage for humankind; without it, shared knowledge and collective action in the world would be much more difficult and probably much less successful.

However, it is the inclusion of two further elements of 'objectivity' that both give us the modern sense of the term and make it more problematic; the notion of objectivity as the erasure of the personal, and the refutation of judgement, idiosyncrasy or values in the production of scientific knowledge. Like other elements of objectivity, this self-restraint on the part of scientists is something that is done; it is a form of (self) orientation, which Daston calls 'aperspectival objectivity'. It derives from the understanding that experiential information about the world is relational; that is, it reflects both the properties of the phenomenon being experienced and the person experiencing it. Objectivity, as restraint and self-effacement, attempts to get at the 'really real', to record the properties of things without the 'contaminating' influence of vagaries of individual perception or judgement that come with epistemological subjectivity. This concern lies behind the methodological preference for strict procedural rules for measurement and recording, preferably executed using technological means. The ideal of 'mechanical objectivity' derives from the perceived incorruptibility of the mechanical:

> it was a nineteenth century commonplace that machines were paragons of certain human virtues [...] patient indefatigable machines would relieve human workers whose pace slackened, whose hands trembled. Scientists praised automatic recording devices and recorders in much the same terms [...] the fact that machines had no choice but to be virtuous struck scientists distrustful of their own powers of self-discipline as a distinct advantage. Instead of freedom of will, machines offered freedom from will.
>
> *(Daston and Galison 1992, p83)*

There is, again, a certain logic and utility in this. Empirical measurements of phenomenon, whether complex or simple, are more likely to be accurate if they are made with care and attention and checked rather than deriving from a loose, careless or off-hand observation. As the practice of science grew from relatively small, self-contained communities of knowledge, where most people knew each other on a personal basis, to a more dispersed, global community where personal relations were not guaranteed and conducting science relied increasingly on large networks of people, with varying skill levels, to make observations, collect specimens and samples from far flung corners of the globe, and quantify populations and phenomena for scientists to study (Livingstone 2003), it became increasingly important to impose shared, agreed-upon rules, procedures, standards of practice and instruments of measurement to increase the reliability and trustworthiness of reported data. Theodore Porter (1995) has argued that one of the reasons numbers, and quantified information, has such authority – even ubiquity – in the modern world, is that numbers travel well. Specifically, once a basic scheme of symbols and meanings of numeracy is widely established, "[f]or people who don't know one another, don't live near each other, don't share similar backgrounds, or don't trust one another, numbers can ease communication, coordinate activities, and settle disputes" (Espeland 1997, p1109).

This is partly because numbers reduce the messiness of real phenomena in the world to a discrete figure. Quantification strips out context, removing 'extraneous' detail to give a communicable piece of information whose clarity and meaning is less open to contestation than an oral or written account. All systems of measurement discipline the measurer to some degree, reducing their discretion and judgement by imposing procedural rules for how the measurement should be made and communicated, but quantification excels at it. Quantified data, being abstracted par excellence, is also very detachable from specific situations, able to be transmitted, stored, combined, and enrolled in calculations. They also allow large complex phenomena like populations to be reduced to manageable sets of information. This is particularly evident in the use of quantified measurements by nation states to understand, and control, their territory and populations through official statistics, censuses, and categories (Scott 1998). Indeed, Porter has argued that the use of quantification spread from state bureaucracies into the scientific realm, not the reverse, as a response to the growth and internationalisation of science. Quantification and depersonalisation are useful strategies for creating shared, empirical public knowledge when personal connections are absent and scientists did not necessarily trust each other's reports or claims. In these domains, both political and scientific, where trust and legitimacy were at stake, quantification provided an attractive solution.

However, problems come from the conflation of the different meanings of 'objectivity' and the expansion of this stance of 'aperspectival objectivity' to imply that true knowledge about the nature of things (the 'really real') is producible through, sufficiently disciplined, value-free mechanical measurement of, preferably quantified phenomena and only by this method. There is a difference between (rightly) rejecting the idea that scientists can or should change results to suit what they would prefer to be true, to embracing the conceit of a 'view from nowhere', the idea that researchers – or indeed anyone making empirical claims about the world through measuring and quantifying phenomena – comes to the work with no assumptions, no prior commitments or values, that they expunge all trace of themselves from the practice of producing knowledge. Instead, it is important to recognise that there are always, inescapably choices and judgements involved in any empirical exercise. There is the choice of what to measure in the first place; deciding which features best define a phenomenon depends at least in part on *why* we want to measure that phenomenon in the first place. The adequacy of the method and means of measurement thus depends on the reasons for measuring. In practice, it is often the case that considerations of what can already be done, and especially what can be done relatively quickly and affordably, informs the choice of parameters and the means of assessing a phenomenon, an approach which Hogle (2009) describes as 'pragmatic objectivity'. Then there is the choice of units. The forms in which any measurement is communally expressed are somewhat arbitrary. A centimetre is not truer or more real a measure than an inch or indeed a cubit. Any unit of measurement is an intermediary that represents nothing but its own value (Vincent 2022). It is also necessarily an abstraction, a representation of certain selected features of a phenomenon at the expense of others. There is then, no such thing as 'raw data'; the concept is an oxymoron, as all data is the result of prior decisions and actions about what, how, when, and where to measure, how to format and store the information that results from measuring, and what to exclude, as well as include (Gitelman and Jackson 2013). Indeed, to be useful data, especially digital data, needs metadata – that is data about the data – describing how, when, and sometimes why the information was produced. Even machines do not truly replace judgement. Every measuring device, however automated, digitised, and so on, was designed by people to function in a certain way, to certain specifications, with certain choices and judgements made in the design process. Thus, choice and judgement are not eliminated merely displaced in the production of knowledge. Thirdly, and no less importantly there is the interpretation of information, another juncture at which judgement inescapably enters. Data is never 'self-evident' – it does not speak for itself and must be 'made to speak' by interpreting and giving it meaning. Often this meaning depends on the context in which the information was generated, especially where acts of measuring and counting are informed by prior theorisation about the nature of the phenomenon under examination, and by the purposes for which the data was generated:

> Data too need to be understood as framed and framing, understood, that is, according to the uses to which they are and can be put. Indeed, the seemingly indispensable misperception that data are ever raw seems to be one way in which data are forever contextualized — that is, framed — according to a mythology of their own supposed decontextualization.
>
> *(Gitelman and Jackson 2013, p5–6)*

Again, there are issues of power and judgement; who has the authority to interpret data and which interpretations become durable and legitimated?

Thus, there are several inescapable choices involved in measuring and quantifying. The first is what to measure; how to define a phenomenon so that it is amenable to assessment, and equally which features are not worth capturing, what information should be discarded. This is even more true in relation to quantification, where most of the 'messiness' of the totality of heterogeneous qualitative information available about a phenomenon must be stripped out to reduce it to a quantified figure. The second choice relates to which unit or scale to use, as there will always be multiple ways of dividing up any natural or social phenomenon. Here the metaphor of the map is useful. A map is informed by data about phenomena that exist independently of us (are ontologically objective), derives from empirical assessment of that phenomenon and makes it communicable (is epistemologically objective), but is necessarily still a selective representation.

A map that is the same scale as the terrain it maps is effectively useless. Any mapmaker must decide what purpose the map is to serve (a globe, for example is no use for local travel planning) and which features to include and which to exclude. The third element of judgement concerns the interpretation of the information generated, what it means and how to respond to it. None of these questions is resolvable by appeal to nature alone, but is always a matter of (social) power, convenience, tradition, or persuasiveness; in other words a human decision. The 'really real' – knowledge independent of any mind – is impossible, a modernist mirage that can never be obtained. None of this is to say that we should not measure and quantify phenomena such as bodies, symptoms, behaviours, and traits, or to enrol this information in schemes of classification and calculation in our quest to treat disease and alleviating suffering. These are all important tools for understanding and shaping our material and social environment. Rather, the point is to employ them with a degree of (epistemic) humility, to recognise that data can only ever be a partial account of the world, that it is always a mediation of reality, the map rather than the territory. As the next section will show, in medicine, as elsewhere, measurement is an activity with consequences and it matters which maps of the world we draw.

Classification, representation, and consequence

Since much of personalised medicine is about more refined, more stratified diagnosis of patient populations, it is pertinent now to turn to the role of measurement and categorisation in diagnosis. Diagnosis can be considered in terms of classification, process, and consequence (Jutel and Nettleton 2011). Classification, in that diagnosis constitutes the categories and labels that make up the officially recognised list of diseases and medically-recognised problems at any given time. Process refers to the activity of assigning an individual to one or other pre-existing category of diseases, usually by measuring and counting various symptoms, behaviours, and physical or biochemical signs. The consequences that flow from diagnosis include access (or not) to healthcare and resources, attaining a label that legitimates what might otherwise be considered social deviance as 'sickness', and marks that patient as a set of data points and information that can travel to other contexts and form part of an evidence base informing treatment, guiding research, and feeding back into appraisal of medical services among other uses. There is a feedback loop here; new research means new measurements and new classifications, which in turn change the experiences and identities of patients, medical professionals, models of treatment, and indeed the formal classification of diseases.

To give a historical example, consider the development of modern techniques for measuring growth and height, especially applied at scale. Technologies of measurement, in this case, the stadiometer and growth chart, play a key role in establishing medical authority over physical states by transforming qualitative descriptions into quantitative assessments, transferring authority for knowing symptoms from the (epistemologically) subjective account of the patient to the objective, empirical knowledge of the medical professional. In the early part of the nineteenth century, Villermé and Quetelet (see Chapter 1) had already begun the application of statistical means to study the effects of living conditions on health, primarily assessed through measurement of physical characteristics including height and weight (Tanner 1981). A new tradition of national and regional growth studies appeared, born of the reaction of humanitarians to the appalling conditions of the poor and of their children. The first British factory report, published in 1833, drew upon the public health work of Villermé and Quetelet comparing the height of factory-employed children to the statistical average height for their age groups as an indicator of overall health status (Tanner 1981). Growth, as a major component of child health, was also monitored through the spread of school-based height surveys in Europe and America. The basis of diagnosis, and medical authority, begins with the measurement and comparison of individuals against the group or population and their subsequent categorisations as 'normal' or 'abnormal' usually through applying statistical conventions (Jutel 2011). Of course, extremes of human stature had been recognised for centuries as 'dwarves' or 'giants', but the instrumental measurement of height, bone age, and fat distribution, and the calculation of growth rates at the population level, meant that people – especially children – could now be scientifically classified as 'abnormally' short or tall, based on statistical cut-off points. Abnormal short stature, for example, being considered height two standard deviations and more below the population average adjusted for age and sex (Hall 2006).

Quantifying growth brought into being new diagnostic categories, and new 'types' of person: it was now possible to be identified as 'abnormally short' or 'abnormally tall' and to have this as part of one's medical and to an extent one's personal identity. First, abnormal stature became a quantifiable symptom that could be used in emerging diagnostic categories. In 1938, Henry H. Turner had published a report describing characteristic symptoms of reduced growth, sexual infantilism and developmental abnormalities, which became known as Turner's syndrome (Medvei 1993). In 1937, Fuller Albright described a syndrome of hormone-related precocious sexual development in females that also resulted in reduced stature (Albright's Syndrome) and in 1942 characterised Klinefelter's Syndrome, which causes excessive height in boys. Later, hormone-based treatments for abnormal stature were developed; human growth hormone to boost height in abnormally short children, and oestrogen or testosterone to stunt the growth of respectively female or male children with predicted abnormally tall stature (Lee and Howell 2006; Tattersall 1996). Here we see a familiar slippage from stature as a diagnostic measure, to stature as something to be treated in its own right.

This example shows how the conflation of different meanings of 'objectivity' can be misleading. The children in the factory and school surveys were real, and their height was an ontologically objective feature of their material bodies. Empirically measuring and charting the range of height measurements brought this information into legibility as shared, epistemologically objective information. The choice of plus or minus two standard deviations from the normal (average) height as the cut-off point between normal and abnormal stature certainly appears more aperspectivally objective, more detached and impersonal, than for example a physician's individual preference about what was or was nor a healthy height, because it employs a statistical convention, widely shared by an expert community and developed 'elsewhere'. However, standard deviation as a tool for distinguishing normal from abnormal still ultimately relies on the assumption that the distribution within a population of a characteristic like height not only does, but also *should*, mimic the normal curve. The statistical norm – that is the population average – comes to have a normative weight. It very readily becomes positioned as the desirable, the 'natural' or healthy state, providing a rationale for medical intervention. This is true for characteristics such as height, weight, and often for physical appearance as well (Parens 2006). In practice, even this degree of detachment was not always achievable: treatment records show that what was considered 'too tall' for girls was often a predicted height taller than the male average, and that often hormone treatment for short boys and tall girls was often considered with the aim of attaining 'a more socially acceptable height' (Morrison 2015).

From this example, we can see how the statistical categories created by measurement of populations (and phenomena) can segue from being abstract denominations that analysts use to understand populations to being identities that people inhabit, and which gain a social reality, as they become the basis for acting and organising social relations. Moreover, we can see how new measurements, and the categories they create can come to discipline the subjects of those categories as well. Once a person comes under the medical authority through a diagnosis or label, there is an accompanying injunction for the sick to get well, the abnormal to attain normality. This is clearly an issue of normative judgement, it is not something that can simply be said to 'be there' in the data, but nor would it be possible without the legibility of traits that measurement and (diagnostic) categorisation makes possible. Diagnosis thus simultaneously transforms the individual (the personal biography and meanings of illness in a person's life) and links to the professional and institutional (the organisation of clinical medicine and the roles, responsibilities, education, and expertise of healthcare professionals) and the societal (data about rates and prevalence of diagnoses and lifetime outcomes feed into the administrative, bureaucratic, and statistical systems of national states to model and plan for resource allocation, public health, and so on, and also inform research funding and clinical trials).

Disease categories are not fixed but vary over time. The history of disease classification is both a historical record of how disease has been defined and what characteristics and traits particular societies have considered worthy of pathologising over time (Blaxter 1978). As noted, there is always a choice of what to measure and why. Height and growth became socially important at a particular time under particular circumstances in nineteenth century Western Europe. The same has been true of many other human traits and behaviours in particular times and places. It is also possible for traits to be removed from the register of the pathological, the expunging of homosexuality as a mental disorder from the Diagnostic and Statistical Manual of Mental Disorders (DSM) being a prime example of how changing social values impact the boundaries and focus of medical authority over time. Although this iterative flux of diagnostic categories over time is recognised, some personalised medicine initiatives aim for a more radical set of changes, rapidly influencing multiple diagnostic categories, which brings its own problems. As Green et al explain,

> Personalization is dependent on the ability to identify similar patients, which presupposes continuity in the (historical) health records and across sites.

> Yet, the aim of a *highly dynamic taxonomy* risks undermining existing practices of data generation and validation, and thereby the very data that personalized diagnostics need.
>
> *(2022, p7 emphasis added)*

There is an inherent paradox in the idea of a perpetually fluid, updating classification of disease that is still founded on correlations with historic data sets that use stable classifications of disease derived from standardised practices of measurement and assessment. If the gradual flux of diagnostic categories over time becomes a digitally driven churn, there are no guarantees that the new and existing means of measurement will all align to produce coherent new categories. This can be illustrated with some examples from genetics and genomics.

Genetics, as we have already glimpsed in relation to pharmacogenomics, is another powerful tool for dividing and classifying human populations. The application of genetics, and genomics, to diagnosis and (re)classification of disease, as well as to categorisation of human traits, has significant power to challenge or reframe existing categories that people use to make sense of themselves and their identities, and sometimes give rise to entirely new ones. This is particularly potent due to the cultural power of 'the gene' as the perceived 'blueprint for life', the molecular basis for appearances, traits, and even behaviours. In the early stages of the Human Genome Project, social scientists were concerned that the reframing of many common illnesses in terms of their genetic causes would promote a reductionist and determinist view of human health and disease: you have gene 'x' and therefore you have disease 'y', regardless of environmental or social determinants of health (Nelkin and Lindee 1995; ten Have 2001). However, the reality has proved rather more complex. Genes are only ever one index of measurement in the diagnostic process. Indeed, as noted above, genetic information often relies for its meaning on correlation with other health information, such as phenotype (physical manifestations of pathology) and disease progression, as well as other biomarkers and physical or chemical indicators of pathology. However, these different measurements do not always align in practice: not everyone with gene 'x' has symptom 'y' or trait 'z'. This is the case with Rhett's Syndrome, for example, a rare disease with a characteristic phenotype. The development of a monogenetic test for Rhett's revealed that some children with the classic Rhett's phenotype did not have the Rhett's gene variant, while other patients who did have the 'correct' gene had very different, non-characteristic phenotypic symptoms. In this case, the final diagnosis is a matter of professional medical judgement about which diagnostic category will be most useful for the patient in directing future treatment (Featherstone and Atkinson 2011). Latimer et al (2006) report a similar situation in their study of the production of genetic diagnoses in cases of childhood dysmorphia. They highlight the different types of 'seeing work' involved in interpreting the multiple, technologically mediated inputs such as genetic test results, scans, patient histories, and biomarker profiles. These results, scans and other data, do not speak for themselves but are, and indeed must be, interpreted by different experts in diagnostic team meetings. This exercise of clinical judgement requires as much tacit skill, based on experience and practice, as it does recourse to formulaic assessment and evidence-based guidelines. These interactions, where diagnosis is made, represent "the micropolitics of medical knowledge, where the personalised authority of the clinician intersects with and may overrule knowledge invoked on the basis of research and journal science" (Latimer et al 2006, p604).

Expanding genetic knowledge from targeted genes, or panels of genes, to larger tracts of genomic data can also introduce further uncertainties. Clinical genome sequencing is usually undertaken with a specific diagnostic question in mind. Due to the correlative nature of genetic data, results can be separated into a number of categories; those results that related to genes whose variants have a known association with the condition, or suspected condition, in question; results about gene variants where the gene in question is not immediately relevant to the clinical question; and variants of unknown significance (VUS). The latter two examples show how more data does not always automatically mean a more refined or more certain diagnosis. Genomic results on variants not deemed immediately relevant to the clinical question at hand are variously termed incidental, accidental, secondary, unsolicited, unexpected, unrelated, non-pertinent, ancillary, and additional findings. VUS are those variants in genes where there is insufficient data to know what significance, if any, they may have for the diagnosis. There has been considerable debate, and no little controversy, about whether genomics health services around the world should return incidental findings and VUS to patients, and to date different countries have pursued different approaches (Morrison et al 2020). Moreover, the distribution of genetic (un)certainty is not equal across populations. The majority of genetic (GWAS) and genomic research has recruited participants from white, Caucasian populations in high-income countries (Hindorff et al 2018; Landry et al 2018). This has been an issue since the first pharmacogenetic tests (Currie et al 2006) and continues to be an issue. This means that the correlations that give genetic variants meaning are often less robust for non-Caucasian populations, and the results of genetic tests less reliable and clinically useful in these populations. There have been several calls for more data to increase the representativeness of information used to calculate genetic associations. However, increasing 'diversity' in genomic (or other) data is not simply about increased data harvesting; it requires consideration of how diversity is configured; geographical, ethnic, by age or sex, by environmental exposure, lifestyle, etc., and what kind(s) of diversity are relevant to the research question at hand (Global Alliance for Genomics and Health 2024). Moreover, many historic attempts to acquire genetic data from indigenous populations have been designed to extract data in ways that add value to the collectors (often through ownership or intellectual property rights|) while delivering no tangible benefit to the communities of origin, so it is important to consider ways to embed equity in future attempts to increase the diversity of genomic data and improve the reliability of tests.

Genomic data has also spilled over as a measurement used in a variety of medically-adjacent areas, such as establishing paternity and relatedness, ancestry tracing, and providing nutritional, and lifestyle advice based on genetic markers. Many of these tests are not administered by healthcare professionals but are available 'direct to consumer' via online sales (see also Chapter 4). As with healthcare professionals incorporating genetics into their diagnostic assessments, patients and laypeople also use their own existing knowledge about family history, beliefs about diet, health, lifestyle, and identity to interpret the results of direct-to-consumer genetic tests and make them meaningful within the contexts of their lives and health choices (Harris et al 2016). One particularly challenging aspect of genetic discourses is their potential to ground existing ideas of racial difference in a biological basis. Consider for example, BiDil, a treatment for congestive heart failure whose application was limited by the US medicines regulator, the Food and Drug Administration (FDA) to African American patients only. Although there was no genetic test associated with BiDil, it was associated with personalised medicine and pharmacogenetics because "scientific and popular accounts [...] implicated genetic explanations for the efficacy of the drug in African Americans" (Tutton et al 2008, p465). Again, deterministic approaches to data meet the indeterminacy of complex real social situations. How physicians and prospective patients came to an agreement about who was 'really' African-American (a social not a biological category) was in practice a somewhat fraught process of negotiation (Braun et al 2007). Beyond this, genetic tests of 'ancestry' have been invoked in disputes about tribal membership and belonging (TallBear 2013), ethnic community membership, and even White nationalism (Panofsky and Donovan 2019). Part of the problem is that 'ancestry' is a nebulous term with different meanings that often span and conflate social and genetic meanings; for example, 'African ancestry' often simultaneously merges geographic and racial identifiers onto biological markers (Global Alliance for Genomics and Health 2024). Again, with practices of (genetic) measurement, the categories that are brought into being represent an abstraction of the reality they purport to capture:

> For an individual, their genetic ancestry is then defined as the subset of paths through their family tree through which they have inherited DNA from specific ancestors. It is possible to produce coarse summaries of the information in this human family tree in various ways, for example by allocating each individual to one or a percentage of more than one group. These abstractions have the disadvantage that they risk essentializing genetically defined groups, when we know that human genetic variation varies in a continuous fashion.
>
> *(Global Alliance for Genomics and Health 2024, p6–7)*

It is very rare that genetic ancestry claims are determinative; the outcomes of disputes and reception of such claims typically depends on the context of discussion, the alignment or divergence from other types of claim (for example claims based on family history or tribal sovereignty) and other social factors. Genetic tests do not ultimately settle issues of racial and group identity but they have, perhaps irrevocably, become a mediating factor in such disputes.

The algorithmic age and the futures of personalised medicine

The final section of this chapter turns to the futures in, and of, personalised medicine. The concept of data-driven personalised medicine is intimately bound up with futurity. It is, as discussed in Chapter 1, a set of promissory discourses, optimistic about the future benefits of digitisation and personalisation in healthcare. The big data element of PM is also bound up with 'future value' and with prediction, that is, with calculating futures. Diagnostic inferences about present conditions drawn from data can also be extended to prognosis about disease progression and treatment outcomes, and extrapolated to consider lifetime risk of developing a disease or condition. This, again, is not wholly novel. The insurance industry has always been built on correlating sociodemographic detail with mortality statistics, but again precision medicine represents an intensification of the scope and scale of data used to inform calculations. In part risk prediction has been criticised for bringing into being the category of the healthy but 'at risk' person – not a patient but potentially, and perhaps enduringly a "patient in waiting" (Timmermans and Buchbinder 2010). At issue is the notion that if someone is predicted, on the basis of a genetic variant or biomarker to have a 20% lifetime risk of 'disease x', this is based on data that shows that of every one hundred people for whom data is available, and who have the relevant gene variant or biomarker, 20 will develop the disease at some point in their lifetime and 80 will not. Which category any individual person falls into is fundamentally unknowable until either they manifest the disease or they die (i.e. retrospectively). But, as will be discussed in Chapter 4, the preventive element of P4 (predictive, preventive, personalised, and participatory) medicine can include a normative injunction to act on risk (another case of a measure disciplining its subjects) and can be used as a device to entice people into greater healthcare consumerism. A great deal of contemporary data collection and creation of data intensive infrastructures (see next chapter) is driven by the perception that it can yield as-yet-unknown and unspecified patterns and correlations:

> Proponents of precision in multiple policy domains predicate claim its value lies in both its future value as new associations are made visible through various automated analytics. This *displacement into the future* is key to the speculative political economy of data whereby assumed future use and exchange value is presented as the justification for gathering data in the present.
>
> *(Kuch et al 2020, p528 emphasis added)*

The 'value' at stake here is both use value (utility) and monetisable value. The latter is presently evident, while the former often remains speculative – a reminder that data-driven personalised medicine is also, and always, a business model (Crawford et al 2014; Reimann et al 2012).

Such speculative data mining is underwritten by the idea, introduced earlier, that sufficient volumes of data alleviate the need for research questions or theories (for example theories of disease categorisation and causation) entirely:

> Big Data analytics are built on the premise that data should not be collected and used for a specific purpose or reason, but rather that they should be relentlessly collected, stored, used, and reused to find patterns, statistical correlations, and to create group profiles. The purposes for their collection, their actual uses, and understanding of their value only come after the fact.
>
> *(Dove and Ozdemir 2015, p18)*

However, as a large part of this chapter has been dedicated to illustrating, this idea that data can be fully decontextualised, and 'raw' or purified from the circumstances of its generation is an illusion. In personalised medicine, as in other precision fields, data is always the product of strategies of measurement, of the affordances of instruments of measurement, of the context(s) and rationale of its generation, and of the contingencies of historical record keeping. Data available for calculations also depends on the sociotechnical infrastructures that enable data flows and mediate access, and on the legal and regulatory frameworks that govern the collection, use and reuse of information, especially personal medical and biological information (see Chapter 6). The ethos of collecting data for as yet unknown purposes is especially problematic for privacy, and where personal data is concerned, runs counter to the principle of data minimisation enshrined in legislation such as the EU General Data Protection Regulation (GDPR).

Increasingly, as attested to in the quote from Kuch et al (2020), the volumes of data required for personalised medicine necessitate some degree of automation to effect computational analysis, often in the form of artificial intelligence. 'Artificial Intelligence', which some consider the future of data-driven medicine, is a widely used, but poorly defined term. Taken broadly it can apply to everything from fairly basic algorithms for enacting particular calculations to more advanced technologies like machine learning, neural networks and large language models which can adapt how they process data and make connections between data points based on feedback over time; that is they are to an extent 'learning systems'. AI, in healthcare, as in other domains, is associated with a long list of potential benefits and an equally extensive list of challenges and problems (Aquino et al 2025; Fenech et al 2018; Goirand et al 2021; Morley et al 2020). The latter include issues of ensuring fairness, avoiding bias and discrimination, accuracy, trustworthiness, protecting privacy, and many others. Given the previous two sections of this chapter, which have endeavoured to demonstrate why data can never be simply a perfect mirror of reality, and why measurement, classification, and interpretation are inescapably value-laden processes, this should not be surprising.

All AI must be trained on existing data, data that even in healthcare, represents sedimented prior classifications and assumptions about the world, and often also records of human choices and behaviours. Moreover, AI tools must be *taught* to classify phenomena, which usually requires annotation of examples by humans, and may be reinforced by manual feedback on examples of attempted classification by the AI tool as it iteratively develops a pattern recognition capacity. Often this work is underpaid and done by marginalised or low socioeconomic status groups, but for the purposes of this chapter the main issue is that, as with the design of other instruments of measurement, there is still a strong element of human judgement and choice in the development process. Chapter 1 introduced the example of an algorithm in the US that used reported healthcare costs as a proxy for medical need, and as such, AI systematically underestimated the level of need of black patients (Ledford 2019). This happened because firstly the existing dataset on which the AI was trained was based on a record of biased human practice. The data were an accurate report of medical decisions that had been made, but they were not neutral. If an AI system takes past data as a model for how future data should look, then human bias, prejudice or neglect recorded by existing datasets will be replicated and projected as the predicted (or worse, desired) state of future affairs. Secondly, the choice of healthcare costs as a proxy measure for medical need was a design choice by the AI developers, who assumed an equality of representativeness across ethnic groups where none existed.

As noted above statistical analysis of data can create new categories of people and phenomena, with very real social effects. Another element of these categorisations of the world is that the bureaucrat or statistician's model of the world is invariably an impoverished one compared to the reality of lived experience (Scott 1998). Measurement, especially when quantified, necessarily operates by reducing and excluding information in order to create a manageable, malleable representation of the world. The information that is excluded often pertains to those aspects of the world, and to those characteristics of people and communities, that are already marginalised, and which may not even be visible to those doing the classification. People with excluded traits thus become 'anomalous' or illegible in the dominant classifications, itself a form of harm, but one that can also lead to greater and very material harms of injustice, exclusion and persecution. The same is true when pattern recognition and classification is outsourced to algorithmic systems:

> In creating and advancing algorithmic recommendation and decision-making systems, designers consolidate and ossify power, granting it to AIs under the false belief that they *necessarily* make better or even more informed decisions. Part of the harm surfaces when the data or the code, or both, go uninterrogated before and during deployment. But part of the harm emerges later, as these

> systems impose the worldview instantiated by the "abridged maps" of the world they generate.
>
> *(Alkhatib 2021, p2 emphasis in original)*

This is particularly egregious when AI systems are used to predict future behaviour and health statuses.

AI systems have been promoted as being able to infer a wide range of social and behavioural traits, including employability, sexuality, voting preferences, and numerous others and outcomes based on data on bodily characteristics such as gait or facial structure (Stark and Hutton 2021). Such correlations are both spurious and egregious; Stark and Hutton consider them no more than automated phrenology. However, the combination of quantification and mechanical objectivity gives AI a veneer of objectivity, a culturally embedded blindness to the distortions rendered by the AI mirror. This is often exploited by parties with AI systems to sell or promote and can make the choices underpinning its functioning hard to detect, let alone contest, especially when automated systems are rolled out at scale.

If AI is the future, or one of the futures of personalised medicine, it is clear that like big data, it is an extension and application of what has gone before. Some of the critique in this chapter has taken aim at the grand narrative, the totalising vision of universal measurement and calculation, which is of course unrealisable. Many of the examples presented throughout the course of this book will deal with more concrete instantiations of personalised medicine, focused on particular data types, with specific research aims, and more limited aspirations of control and calculation. Nonetheless, the lessons outlined in this chapter still apply. Measuring and quantifying phenomena does not simply represent them but actively constitutes an intervention in the world. Put another way, measurement is not innocent but changes the world it claims to capture and has consequences. The lesson of this chapter is not to reject measurement, nor to abandon quantification and calculation as ways to comprehend the world, but to resist the slippage from recognising that data has something useful to tell us about objective phenomena to believing that it has everything to say. As with diversity in genomic data part of the answer is better data not more data and more attention to equity and social benefit. It is to take care with the maps we draw and not to mistake the map for the territory.

3

INFRASTRUCTURES AND INFRASTRUCTUR-*ING*

Infrastructures are socio-technical arrangements comprising "the basic physical and organizational structures and facilities needed for the operation of a society or enterprise" (Oxford English Dictionary, N.D.). They may involve anything and everything from tangible material components such as roads, buildings, and equipment to intangible elements such as standards, rules, visions, interfaces, symbols, and more. Consider the road network. As part of the transport infrastructure, road networks contain material elements, most obviously the roads themselves, but also regulations in the form of 'rules of the road' that govern how people drive, standards for materials (e.g., tarmac), information (road signs), conduct (speed limits), symbols for communication (road signs again), and interfaces with other infrastructure such as that for pedestrian travel, cycling, fuel provision (petrol stations), subsistence (food and accommodation for long distance travellers such as motorway service stations), and skills (road builders and maintenance workers, drivers). At the same time, road networks are also shaped by normative visions about what they are for and how, and by whom they should be used (heavy goods vehicles for example may be restricted from narrower suburban streets). Many everyday infrastructures, such as roads, or the electricity or water networks are often taken for granted – at least as long as they work (Slota and Bowker 2017). Their critical role in enabling many activities in our everyday lives often only becomes visible when infrastructures either break down, or when aspects of their design exclude us from utilising them such as public spaces without wheelchair access (Star 1999).

As previous chapters have discussed a great deal of personalised medicine (PM) is 'data driven'. As a first step this requires increased datafication, that is, the recording of information of various kinds in digital form. Sometimes this means manually inputting existing physical records, such as medical histories, into digital formats, while a great deal of digital activity is now automatically turned into

DOI: 10.4324/9781003279556-3

electronic data such as online actions (e.g., visiting a website, using an app), or readings from digitally connected devices and smart sensors. In the medical space, this could include medical apps, automatic digitisation of scans and other readings from digitally connected devices such as magnetic resonance imaging machines, or readings from wearable devices connected to the internet. All of this data generation and storage requires infrastructure. It requires interfaces to collect information, whether as signals from equipment or the notes of a healthcare professional typing on a keypad or using a touchscreen device. It requires software modules and standardised protocols to store and access this data, algorithms to process it, classification systems to order and make sense of information, and importantly for PM, information communication technologies to share and aggregate digitised medical data. All of these elements are part of the infrastructure that makes digital data analysis possible.

Infrastructures are also about circulation, about mobilising entities and making them available across distances, whether this is people, resources, power, materials and goods, ideas, or indeed, data (Morrison 2017). Given their intimate relationship with data, infrastructures of PM are also implicated in shaping who or what is counted and therefore comes to count, and who does not (see Chapter 2). Data is, understandably, the focus of most PM infrastructures, although biobanks, stem cell banks and registries follow a longstanding tradition in the life sciences of making standardised (biological) materials available for research as the basis for future knowledge production (Morrison 2017). Even collections of biological materials are to a large degree dependent on integrated digital infrastructure such as online catalogues, and digital shipping trackers to allow the circulation of biological samples (Brown and Williams 2015). Holmberg et al (2011, p742) describe this realm of digital records, and sometimes models, of biological materials as the "bio-virtual": "a specific form of life, which exists as information, data and informational flows".

This brings us to a second key aspect of PM infrastructure development; *platformisation*. Digital platforms, or more accurately, digital platform businesses, are ubiquitous in the contemporary world. Examples include Amazon, Uber, Facebook, and indeed all online purchasing services, social media systems, as well as online financial and security services. Poell et al (2019, p3) define platforms as "(re-)programmable digital infrastructures that facilitate and shape personalised interactions among end-users and complementors, organised through the systematic collection, algorithmic processing, monetisation, and circulation of data". Digital platforms then are a form of (data intensive) infrastructure. *Platformisation* as a term refers to the growing importance, and intersection of platforms in different sectors of life. The penetration of healthcare, medicine and medical research by platforms is constituent of PM. Platforms have important social and economic effects. Platforms enable (medical) data to be configured as an asset, where aggregated data becomes valuable for PM and as a result access can be restricted and rendered contingent on, for example payment or contractual terms (Faulkner-Gurstein and Wyatt 2023).

The distribution of power between platform managers, users and contributors is often decidedly uneven and weighted in favour of managers (Poel et al 2019). Moreover, platforms also produce effects on the cultural practices of users as they adapt and respond to the ways that platforms can enable, incentivise or restrict behaviours.

These infrastructures of PM are the focus of this chapter. The chapter begins by outlining some of the key elements of PM infrastructures and how to think critically about them. Many PM projects are large-scale infrastructure building endeavours. They require considerable investment of time, labour, capital, and resources. Moreover, they are always entangled with varying socio-cultural and political actors and values (Bowker 1994; Green et al 2022; Hogle 2018; Hughes 1993; Latour et al 1986). As such, infrastructure and the work of building, maintaining and connecting infrastructures always has politics, and PM is no different. Here the politics of PM will be examined in terms of how future orientated expectations and visions drive, and shape specific PM infrastructuring projects, and by considering the role of policymaking in setting standards, regulations, and rules that both shape digital and material infrastructure and are themselves a form of intangible infrastructure making. The remainder of the chapter then focuses on two case studies of large-scale PM infrastructure development; the US 'All of US' project, and the recent EU attempts to build 'digital twins' across Europe (European Commission 2023; Precision Medicine Initiative (PMI) Working Group Report to the Advisory Committee to the Director, NIH 2015; Spanish Presidency Council of Europe 2023). Each of these case studies, in different ways, takes a deeper look at the politics of PM infrastructures, from the plurality of competing technological visions for new PM infrastructure projects – each with its own account of what a desirable future should look like and a technological roadmap for how to get there – to the messier business of building and implementing PM infrastructure, where inescapably value-laden decisions shape future research trajectories, engage questions of social justice, access to the benefits of medical research, surveillance, what counts as (good) evidence, who gets to decide, and who is left out of decision-making.

Studying infrastructures

To understand how infrastructures come about, it is important to bear in mind that they are never merely neutral technical arrangements, nor do they come about in a vacuum. Rather, they are shaped to function in specific ways to serve particular societal aims (Pinch and Bijker 1984) that are inseparable from the values and visions of those who shape them (Bowker 1994; Green et al 2022; Hogle 2018; Hughes 1993; Latour et al 1986). Consequently, infrastructure attempts for PM – such as our two case studies – are performative in facilitating or obstructing certain relationships, shaping the way we understand and look at the world (Slota and Bowker 2017).

Infrastructures are neither static nor homogeneous, but a patchwork of fully or partially interconnected systems that are continuously 'in-the-making' to enable specific visions of technological development (Bowker et al 2010; Edwards et al 2009; Felt et al 2020; Grisot and Vassilakopoulou 2017; Lievevrouw 2023; Pipek and Wulf 2009). Recent research refers to infrastructur-*ing,* emphasising this continuous 'in-the-making' aspect – the tinkering, refining, editing, patching, and 'making do' that characterises messy technological development in the real world (Bowker et al 2010; Edwards et al 2009; Felt et al 2020; Grisot and Vassilakopoulou 2017; Lievevrouw 2023; Pipek and Wulf 2009). Both the All of US project and the different EU initiatives for digital twins can be regarded as parts of the ongoing infrastructuring of PM, each shaping the boundaries of PM. Infrastructuring incorporates:

> the *prior work (*be it building, organization, agreement on standards, and so forth), that supports and enables the activity we are really engaged in doing. [It] refers to those systems, technologies, organizations, and built artefacts that do not need to be reconsidered at the start of a new venture.
>
> *(Slota and Bowker 2017, p529 emphasis added)*

'Prior work' can include the development of anything, and everything required to progress innovation; from the development of "a set of agreed-upon rules for the production of (textual or material) objects" such as technical standards, guidelines, or regulations (Bowker and Star 1999, p13) to enabling circulation of materials, finances, and data through future-oriented visions. The latter is operationalised by creating the conditions and the consensus rules among actors that allows the mobilisation of resources such as people (skills), capital, goods, ideas, or indeed, data, across distances and jurisdictions (Morrison 2017). Consider the European Union's *1+ Million Genomes* project's aim to create a pan-European Genomic Data Infrastructure (GDI 2022). Beyond the politics and economics of 'European' genetic identity underlying the GDI, the realisation of GDI itself is only made possible by co-developing the 'set of agreed rules' (standards, export controls, intangible technology transfer agreements, etc.) that allows the mobilisation of vast amounts of data and various other related infrastructural resources across "70 institutes from 24 European countries and 2 international organisations" (Genomic Data Infrastructure 2022). Moreover, 'new' infrastructuring endeavours typically build upon an 'installed base' of older existing material and cognitive infrastructures. By incorporating the strengths and limitations of that base, they are therefore also hard to undo (Star and Ruhleder 1994, p113). The infrastructuring of PM serves as a case in point, as we will illustrate in the following sections how the launch of the All of US cohort and the new Virtual Human Twins (VHTs) initiative continues to build on the historical socio-technical entanglement of PM with Big Data aspirations.

Infrastructures and the role of *visions*

As mentioned in the previous section, the 'prior work' of infrastructuring can take different forms. One cluster of ways for the 'doing' of infrastructuring is through expectations and future-oriented visions. Jasanoff and Kim (2015) developed the notion of 'sociotechnical imaginaries', or "collectively held and performed visions of desirable futures" that are derived from "shared understandings of forms of social life and social order attainable through, and supportive of, advances in science and technology" (p19), revealing the intricate relation between political authority and the shaping of science and technology (policies). Since then, the concept has been widely adopted to explore how such future-oriented imaginaries around personalised, digital (health) technologies are embedded in a constantly evolving network of material, social, political, and cultural elements. In line with this, Mager and Katzenbach (2021) argue that sociotechnical imaginaries, though institutionally stabilised, are increasingly shaped by tech companies, turning them into multiple, contested, and commodified visions rather than monolithic, linear aspirations for the future.

While sociotechnical imaginaries often reflect stabilised, collectively held visions, other future-oriented concepts – such as 'vanguard visions' (Hilgartner 2015), 'hypes', and expectations (Borup et al 2006) – highlight how less-stable visions articulated by a few powerful actors can be highly performative in shaping early innovation trajectories. Geiger and Gross (2017) and McFall et al (2020) have illustrated how hypes around new digital technologies (e.g., digital health or behaviour-based insurance) have spurred the concomitant making of insurance practices and digital health markets (Geiger and Kjellberg 2021). Similarly, Green et al (2022)'s work on Danish digital infrastructurings demonstrate how visions of 'big data' impose significant changes on healthcare systems (e.g., new forms of evidence standards), underscoring the powerful transformative role of imagined futures – even when they are not yet institutionally embedded.

Realising these promissory visions of emerging science is not limited to envisioning 'new' ways forward but also includes re-imagining and re-shaping existing arrangements. In PM, this has often meant re-imagining existing legal-institutional arrangements for conducting and regulating medical research to overcome organisational impediments to developing desired visions (Mittra 2013). Consider *The Precision Medicine Initiative's* overarching 'longer-term goals' at launch to "create a research cohort of >1 million American volunteers who will share genetic data, biological samples, and diet/lifestyle information, all linked to their electronic health records if they choose" (PMI 2015). This goal, to enable a data infrastructure not only envisions communitarian notions of patient-data sharing for the common good without which the realisation of PM remains unlikely (see, e.g., our discussion in Chapters 4 and 7) but also enables this by re-imagining and reframing structural impediments to this goal in order to overcome them. PMI's goal is to create a 'new' data repository (infrastructure) that sits separate from yet draws on existing legal institutional arrangements (for informed consent and patient privacy that privilege the individual in medical research) and at once overcomes organisational impediments to the widespread and wide-ranging use of patient data by re-imagining existing structures for organising medical research. In this way, infrastructures performatively produce the conditions and processes that realise certain technological visions instead of others (Butler 1988), shaping futures in specific ways (Slota and Bowker 2017).

Infrastructures and the role of policymaking

A different form of infrastructural work resides in the development of technical standards, guidelines and rules, or regulations. Prior work, especially in the context of setting up 'agreed rules' – whether standards, regulations, or guidelines – is the bedrock upon which innovation processes proceed (Faulkner 2009a). Their centrality to innovation cannot be overestimated even though they are often taken for granted or perceived as external to the core task of infrastructuring because their development tends to 'lag behind' the material development of innovation (Faulkner 2009a, p638). Consider regulatory standards for safety, quality, and effectiveness in health and medicine. These are the key mechanisms not only for creating a legally sanctioned pathway to market for pharmaceuticals and medical devices but also useful tools for harmonising the spectrum of health and biomedical technologies across jurisdictions, and across sectors (Demortain 2011); and therein crucial to supporting market-orientated innovation and development (Davis and Abraham 2011; Hendrickx 2014).

Infrastructures in general and for PM, in particular, are inherently 'multiple' and diverse (Mol 1999). Infrastructuring can not only be done in different ways (e.g., regulations, standardisation, visions), but can also occur simultaneously within different realities, with each underlying 'installed base' (Star and Ruhleder 1994, p113) bringing its own histories, practices, and values. Jasanoff refers in this regard to the concept of 'political culture' or the "systematic means by which a political community makes binding collective choices" (Jasanoff 2005, p21) to demonstrate how socio-technical imaginaries can take different shapes depending on the political traditions and logics of governance in which they are embedded. The intrinsic challenge and ambition of infrastructuring therefore lies in securing consensus across the multiplicity of actors, interests, values, across the diverse multiple infrastructural strands required to work together to enable a cohesive "space within which differences between technical practices, procedures, and forms have been reduced, or common standards have been established" (Barry 2006, p239). Andrew Barry (2006) called these spaces 'technological zones' and found, through his study of the global oil industry, that these more often than not opened up *new* spaces of contestation between the competing interests and ideas of the variety of stakeholders, standards, legislative initiatives, and funding sources (Barry 2001). The reality of infrastructuring PM is not dissimilar to Barry's 'technological zones'. The case studies below will illustrate how the development and delivery of PM similarly evolve through a continuous process of (value) choices among myriad, interests, goals and visions (Tironi and Valderrama 2021).

Case study 1: the Precision Medicine Initiative: infrastructuring (in)equality?

PMI and all of US

The Precision Medicine Initiative (PMI) is a landmark project in the United States aimed at advancing PM. Launched in 2015 under the leadership of President Barack Obama, the PMI was envisioned as a comprehensive, multi-faceted initiative encompassing various PM efforts within the United States (Minari et al 2018). The core focus of the PMI has been the 'All of US' study, an ambitious programme designed to collect extensive health data from a million U.S. residents over the course of several decades. The central aim of the 'All of US' study is to recruit one million U.S. residents to participate in a long-term cohort study that spans 60 years. Participants are asked to contribute a variety of health-related data (e.g., access to existing electronic medical records, donation of blood or tissue samples for genomic analysis, completion of online surveys covering lifestyle, medication usage, and health status, physical measurements (e.g., height, weight, data from wearable devices for self-monitoring). As a cohort study, data is collected at repeated intervals over time, building a longitudinal picture of health changes across the life-course of participants. Importantly, All of US also returns (selected) data back to participants, including the list of selected actionable findings from genomic data recommended by the American College of Medical Genetics, so it provides a case study of an infrastructure-building project that not only aims to collect data but also aims to provide PM data to patient/participants.

As these features suggest, the All of US study has a strong public health focus, and in its aim of generating large volumes of data to identify combinations of factors that impact health outcomes, while using this information to stratify participants into refined groups to develop future targeted medical interventions, it is clearly also a PM project. The PMI exemplifies how large-scale 'Big Science' projects have been performative in rolling out vast data-collection infrastructures for PM. However, as we will argue below, the tensions that have come along with this initiative have also made visible the questions about equity and participation that are enshrined in the material making of this 'All of US' database.

Promoting inclusivity and representation

A key feature of the 'All of US' study has been its emphasis on inclusivity, particularly in terms of the representativeness of the population in the cohort. Historically, medical research has predominantly focused on certain groups, especially white populations. The Precision Medicine Working Group Report (2015) underscored the need for greater representation of diverse populations in biomedical research:

> As a nation that historically includes indigenous people, people who originally migrated or were brought to this country from different parts of the world, and

> more recent and new migrants from numerous countries, the U.S. benefits from the richness of ancestral diversity. The PMI cohort is intended to be a national resource that will, over time, benefit the entire U.S. population. It will leverage our diversity to provide new insights to factors determining health and disease, as well as prevention and therapeutic strategies. Critically, the PMI cohort will be designed to ensure that people historically underrepresented in biomedical research are included in sufficient numbers to allow robust inferences in these groups.
>
> *(Precision Medicine Working Group 2015, p28)*

This focus on diversity aligns with one of the promises of PM. As Van Hoyweghen and Arden (2021, p569) note "[a]n important promise of PM and the genomic sciences that are constitutive to it remains the advancement of social justice by scientific means, including the idea that genomic technologies provide a solution for health disparities". On the other hand, it is also significant because it represents a recognition and an attempt to address some of the inherent challenges of PM. As discussed in Chapter 2, data sets containing data points that are the result of historic (or current) biases in healthcare (e.g., under-diagnosis of certain conditions in minorities or women), or data sets that are used to make PM calculations for populations whose members are not represented in that dataset (e.g., using a data set derived from mainly white European patients to stratify patient populations in sub-Saharan Africa) can lead to further bias, and to discriminatory outcomes such as inefficient, unsuitable or even harmful care decisions being made. Data is not, however, the only domain in which issues of social justice in PM arise.

PM relies on the participation of individuals who provide their health data and biological samples for research (one of its core 'publics' – see Chapter 4). This assumes an implicit – and sometime explicit – social contract between the participants and the developers of PM programmes. The naming of the 'All of US' cohort is a deliberate evocation of this hoped-for sense of American solidarity. Tutton and Prainsack (2011) identified two primary motivations for participation in PM initiatives. The first of these is altruism, the participants who 'donate' their data for the greater good, for the health benefits that might accrue to other people, including future generations. The second motivation, they term the 'entrepreneurial self'; the participant who agrees to take part in return for getting access to their own data. This presumes having access to one's own data is a 'good' in its own right. As Chapter 4 will discuss in more detail, it aligns with discourses of PM that emphasise individual responsibility to make informed medical and lifestyle choices on the basis of the information provided by PM technologies as 'empowering'. In practice, both aspects of this presumed social contract are problematic.

While PM promises 'patient-focused' care, the actual design of PM programmes often overlooks the social context of patients. In the context of North American PM projects, Rothstein (2017) notes that patients who have low digital literacy, low health literacy or whose first language is other than English may struggle to make any meaningful use of data made available to them by PM projects. Online and other forms of data access often neglect patients with disabilities such as visual impairment and dyslexia. There are also a range of cultural reasons why patients from minority ethnic backgrounds could be disincentivised both from participating in medical research in the first place and from asking questions and having extended interactions with healthcare professionals even when PM data is returned to them. These challenges highlight the fragility of the assumed social contract implicit in both altruistic and enterprising models of PM participation; if neither the participant nor the community they recognise stand to benefit in practical terms from PM, then there is little incentive to participate and little benefit in doing so (Rothstein 2024).

These issues of inclusion and utility are also clearly issues that relate to how PM infrastructures are designed and how they (might) actually operate in practice. Through these challenges, we can clearly see the politics of infrastructuring and how issues of access, fairness, and social justice are indeed infrastructural issues. It not only matters what the infrastructures of PM are designed to do, it matters *how* they are designed, for whom they are designed, and what sort of social contract is actually encoded in this design process (Van Hoyweghen and Aarden 2022).

Addressing barriers to participation

The 'All of US' study has made deliberate efforts to increase the inclusivity of its participant base by oversampling from historically underserved groups such as African Americans, Hispanic Americans, people with low socioeconomic status, and rural populations. This approach is in line with what Epstein (2007) terms the 'inclusion and difference' approach to recruitment. Epstein raised a number of concerns with this approach. As discussed in Chapter 2, the way(s) in which we choose to order and categorise people, populations and diseases is always a strategic one – and one that has consequences. There are always decisions about what, how and when to measure, but once categories become formalised in official bureaucratic or institutional practices and operationalised in everyday use, they start to be treated as social realities rather than useful heuristics for understanding the world.

Efforts to target increased participation in PM by gender, ethnicity, age, sexual orientation, and other sociodemographic descriptors, run the same risk of reifying these categories. This is especially the case when genetic research is involved, as certain genes, traits or diseases become closely associated with particular groups (see the discussion of BiDil for African-American heart failure patients in Chapter 2), so that, for example, being Black (a cultural categorisation) becomes associated with higher risk of heart disease or anaemia (medical and biological designations). It is true that some disease-associated genes *can* be found at statistically higher rates of prevalence in particular, culturally defined, populations, but this is a group level calculation. It does not follow that any given individual in that group is at higher risk; it will depend on whether or not they carry the relevant genetic variant. At best they are 'at risk of being at risk' where a visible trait such as racial or ethnic origin is used as a proxy for an unknown probability of disease risk in the absence of any direct biological evidence. This clearly slides all too readily slides into stigmatisation of a person because of their ethnicity (or gender, age, etc.) and can result in unfair discrimination, the very thing that inclusivity initiative are intended to reduce.

Another concern raised by Epstein (2007) is that the increasingly mandatory inclusivity targets seen in medical research, and particular in PM research (Shim et al 2022), leads to a very instrumental focus on *how* to make recruitment more inclusive rather than considering *why* underserved or marginalised communities might be reluctant or unable to take part in PM projects. In practice, many PM projects in the US use geographic location as a proxy for diversity when recruiting participants (Shin et al 2022). The logic of this runs that if you use recruitment centres in different areas with different populations, diversity of recruitment will naturally follow. This does suggest Epstein's concern that the 'how' of diversification takes precedence over the 'why', despite the availability of sociological and ethical evidence on how best to engage marginalised communities (Kraft et al 2018). In addition, PM projects tend to operationalise recruitment through clinical centres that are already integrated into the infrastructure of biomedical research such as having staff with the necessary skills, electronic health record systems that can digitise data and make it available for reuse, experience with securing local research ethics committee approvals et cetera. This shows how building 'new' infrastructures of PM requires building on the 'installed base' (Bowker and Star 1999) of existing infrastructures of medical research and care – and leads to an inherited politics of (existing) infrastructure. The consequence is that those clinical sites that were historically under-resourced and not set up to conduct medical research, and the populations who use them, remain excluded from much of the new infrastructuring efforts of PM. As Shin et al (2022, p306) observe:

> Once these patterns of funding and partnership are set in motion, they tend to self-perpetuate because of restrictions on research funding being spent on capacity building and because of the time limits imposed by grant funding. As one investigator told us, 'there's so much infrastructure cost to setting up something and building relationships and everything else. And not everyone's going to be able to do that, quite frankly'.

This illustrates another aspect of the politics of PM infrastructure. Much academic PM research is supported by grant funding. Funders are under political pressure to 'get results' fast. This limits the money and time available to upgrade clinical infrastructure, meaning researchers must prioritise recruitment sites that can get 'up and running' quickly.

Despite these common limitations, there is evidence that the 'All of US' study has implemented several measures to address structural and cultural barriers to inclusion. These measures include: providing recruitment information in multiple languages, including Spanish, operating a support centre with telephone and online access, offering multiple consent methods, including video and paper-based options, engaging with institutions that serve underrepresented communities, running focus groups in marginalised communities to gather input, and providing sensitivity training to researchers to address stigmatisation and bias (Ferryman et al 2024; Galasso 2024). These are all ways of infrastructuring that aim to produce fairer, more equitable access to PM and demonstrate how design choices and practices in building infrastructure can be informed by ethical and societal concerns as well as scientific and medical ones. Nonetheless, these infrastructural interventions mainly target barriers to participation in PM research. They do less to address the other side of the bargain of PM; fair and equitable access to the benefits of PM.

In particular, economic barriers remain a considerable challenge to the PM promise of 'better healthcare' for all. While the costs of producing information for PM, for example through whole genome sequencing, have decreased sharply since the earliest days of sequencing, the costs of storing, annotating, analysing and interpreting the data, and providing actionable feedback including educational materials for both physicians and patients, and available genetic counselling have not (Rothstein 2017). Similarly, pharmacogenomic medicines and other targeted therapies are increasingly likely to be biological medicines rather than conventional chemical pharmaceuticals and often come with exceptionally high costs per treatment (something discussed in more detail in Chapter 5). Only a relatively small proportion of US citizens have no health insurance at all, but many insurance plans will not extend to cover the more expensive PM tests or therapies (Galasso 2024). Here is another case where the new infrastructures of PM intersect with the installed base of American health care and medical insurance. Again, this is likely to impact already disadvantaged communities the hardest, an important reminder that, however well intentioned "inclusion in itself does not affect inequities" (Galasso 2024, p74).

Here, it is important to note that while some commentators see this primarily as a problem of the US for-profit healthcare system (Rothstein 2024), barriers to both participation and access to medicines persist in relation to PM projects in healthcare systems with universal coverage, as the infrastructures to deliver PM are likely to be concentrated in urban centres (excluding rural populations) and expensive PM therapies will be subject to Health Technology Assessments (HTA) which restrict access to patients with the most serious conditions and those with private health insurance (for treatments public health systems cannot afford to cover). HTA and its impact on PM therapies are discussed in more detail in Chapter 5.

Ultimately this points to a wider politics of PM infrastructuring, in that while individual PM projects may, to varying extents, try to address some aspects of existing health disparities within populations, overall the rise of PM represents a political choice to invest in expensive new infrastructure projects with uncertain, and potentially unequal, benefits rather than, for example, using the same state funds to support lower technology programmes to improve access to existing healthcare services for disadvantaged and minoritised communities (Reardon 2017). Again, none of this is to suggest that All of US will not produce medical benefits, but that is precisely in examining the infrastructuring work of the study that allows us to make visible the challenges in extending these benefits beyond the population of Americans who are "uncommonly tech savvy, highly health literate, self-directed, information seeking, English fluent, health focused, and well insured" (Rothstein 2017, p277–278).

Case study 2: infrastructuring datafication through digital twins in Europe

Digital or virtual twins refer to "a digital replica or representation of a physical object, process, or service" (Kamel Boulos and Zhang 2021, p1). In health and biomedical contexts, digital twins represent:

> a patient-specific virtual representation of real-world systems or processes, that is built on data-driven or knowledge-driven – most often a combination of both – predictive computer models, and that can be used as a clinical decision-support system, a personal health forecasting tool or as a tool for the development and personalisation of medical products.
>
> *(EDITH Website 2022)*

Simply put, medical digital twins are digital models that can be used to mimic individual patients or parts of their bodies such as a particular organ, metabolic process, or physiological state and predict their responses to different therapies and interventions, disease prognosis, or lifetime risk of diseases. Digital twins are not wholly new and indeed exist in many sectors such as in manufacturing, where they are used to test new product designs for optimal performance before having to commit to making an actual physical object. However, their deployment in the health sector, with the promise of enabling faster and more *precise* predictions of diseases, is considered new and having "great potential in advancing personalised care" (European Commission 2023).

In this section, we turn to two different policy initiatives for digital twins to illustrate the entanglement of these PM infrastructurings with normative vision of data-driven digital healthcare. First, we consider one of the EU's newest policy initiatives – the VHT Initiative – to again illustrate how seemingly new infrastructurings are ultimately built on an 'installed base' (Bowker and Star 1999) and bound up with earlier infrastructuring attempts and normative visions around health and biomedical innovation. As we will argue in the section below, the aim of the VHT Initiative to unite the supposedly 'fragmented ecosystem' of digital twins into one 'big' VHT (EDITH 2022; European Commission 2023) could be understood as a re-articulation of previous infrastructurings around digital health, putting forward the idea that (big) datafication is the only way to overcome the so-called healthcare crisis Europe is facing (Lievevrouw and Felt 2026).

Secondly, in this digital twin case study, we also aim to highlight how infrastructuring attempts – in part because they inherently enact certain values – are always opening new spaces of contestation regarding how various aspects of society *ought* to look like (Barry 2006; Bowker and Star 1999). For this, we turn to the world of regulatory approvals for pharmaceuticals. We demonstrate how the European Medical Agency's attempt to infrastructure PM (digital twins) through experimentation with real-world evidence has opened new discussions around 'expertise' and 'risk' in the context of biomedical innovation.

EU's virtual human twin initiative: 'big' visions or old wine in new 'digital twin' bottles?

On 21 December 2023, the MareNostrum5 supercomputer (MN5) was inaugurated at the Universitat Politècnica de Catalunya in Barcelona as part of the Spanish Presidency of the Council of the European Union. As the world's eighth most powerful supercomputer, MN5 is specifically designed to enhance European medical research and is positioned as 'ideal' for performing "large-scale simulations, such as those used in artificial intelligence (AI), enabling researchers and users to solve problems related to medical research, natural language applications or digital twins" (Spanish Presidency Council of Europe 2023). The high hopes of the MareNostrum5 supercomputer for medical innovation were underscored as the launch served a double purpose. It was simultaneously used as a platform for announcing the 'European Virtual Human Twins Initiative', the EU's newest attempt to infrastructure PM across Europe (European Commission 2023; Spanish Presidency Council of Europe 2023). The VHT initiative (hereafter 'the initiative') aims to use advanced supercomputing and AI to accelerate VHT research and technology development for PM among others.

While the EU Commission website on the VHT Initiative makes only a single mention of 'personalised care', references to 'enabling large AI foundational models', 'collaboration environment', or fighting the 'fragmented ecosystem' reveal substantial parts of the 'installed base' (Star and Ruhleder 1994) on which EU's newest infrastructuring attempt for PM continues to build. Similar to the first genetic databases and biobanks, the VHT can be seen as a new 'Big Science' (Davies et al 2013) project that works not only on developing technical PM infrastructure but in doing so also provides a vessel for specific "epistemic ambitions, funding imperatives, research governance, choice[s] and maintenance of infrastructure" (Davies et al 2013, p386). Similar to previous EU infrastructuring attempts for PM (see, e.g., Lievevrouw and Felt 2026), the expansion of the VHT is legitimised out of a continuous need or 'urgency' for more data to enable a better and more precise understanding of new disease categories (Green et al 2022; Hogle 2016; Tarkkala et al 2019). In doing so, the VHT initiative not only serves as a material enabler for digital twin technologies, but it also simultaneously re-enacts a long-standing normative vision that 'Big data' will provide the solution to Europe's alleged healthcare crisis.

This datafication vision – which is reflected in numerous prior EU initiatives related to digital health (see Felt et al 2009; Hoeyer 2016; Hogle 2016; Lievevrouw 2023) – assumes that the best way to comprehend the human body in its fullest granularity is by aggregating as many sources of data as possible to obtain a complete picture of the different diseases and their variations between people. Following this datafication perspective, we must build large data sets and soft- and hardware that are powerful enough to run such complex analytics. Consequently, with its 'big' vision, the VHT Initiative follows a long list of PM infrastructurings enacting the normative assumption "that bigger will be faster, and that faster is better" (Davies et al 2013, p387). Hoeyer (2016) conceptualised this 'need' for more and faster data in healthcare as 'data-intensive resourcing'. He uses this to refer to the various "attempts at getting more data, of better quality, on more people. Sourcing is a dynamic process of creating, collecting, curating, and storing data while simultaneously making them available for multiple purposes, including research, governance and economic growth" (Hoeyer 2016, p73). Or as Hogle (2016) puts it, the idea of "[p]recision medicine is a paragon of big data medicine" (Hogle 2016, p398).

Building on Hoeyer's (2016) definition, three elements are particularly interesting to understand the VHT Initiative as a *new-but similar* infrastructuring of PM: 'more data', on 'more people', for 'multiple purposes'. While the first PM initiatives focused primarily on the creation of large datasets for genomic medicine, over the years this 'big' vision has been widened to include different types of data that could provide a more comprehensive understanding of the interaction between individuals and their environments (Hogle 2016; Tarkkala et al 2019; and see Chapter 2). Consequently, investments have been made not only in the digitisation of medical data (e.g., e-health infrastructures), but also in the interoperability of these different 'big' datasets, and this even beyond the remits of health and care (Lievevrouw 2023). When collecting alternative – social media, lifestyle, or consumer – data, the 'big' data-driven vision has also turned its eye to 'more people', and accordingly has included data collection from healthy citizens (Hogle 2016; Minari et al 2018). Felt et al (2009) speaks in this context of the 'not-yet patient', or how these EU 'big' data policy initiatives enact a specific 'citizen-patient' who has the potential to become a patient at any time, something returned to in Chapter 4.

With the launch of the VHTs initiative the future-oriented 'big' data-driven vision has thus once again boosted the promise of PM in Europe. While the notion of PM is hardly mentioned, a closer look at the Twins initiative reveals however how it continues to build on the historical socio-technical entanglement of PM with Big Data aspirations, therefore turning old 'Big Data' wine into new 'digital twin' bottles.

Digital twins for the 'real-world' quality and safety assessment of personalised medicines in Europe

On 20 September 2022, the European Medical Agency published a favourable qualification opinion for the use of Unlearn.AI's TwinRCT solution, allowing digital twins to potentially be used for narrowing down the selection of trial participants in phases II and III clinical drug trials in Europe. The agency publishes these opinions as a scientific endorsement of a novel methodology that has proven to be promising for the research and development of new pharmaceuticals. This particular EMA publication was regarded with considerable scrutiny as it was the first time ever for a regulatory body worldwide to provide formal support for using machine learning to reduce sample size in pivotal trials (Businesswire 2022). This favourable opinion forms an important element in EMA's recent infrastructure attempts to make room for digital (personalised) technologies within the world of regulatory sciences in Europe. These infrastructuring attempts manifest as the EMA's efforts to develop 'real-world evidence' frameworks for the quality and safety assessment of pharmaceuticals.

This search for alternative forms of evidence has its origins in dissatisfaction with existing standards for quality and safety assessment. When drugs and medical devices are brought to market in Europe, companies are obliged to obtain quality and safety approval from the European Medical Agency (EMA, for drugs) or national regulatory authorities and notified bodies (for medical devices). The 'gold standard', according to the tenets of Evidence Based Medicine, for gathering evidence to proof the quality and safety of medical products is to go through several stages of randomised control trials (RCTs). However, considering the recent rise of personalised medical interventions, this evidence-based method has become increasingly criticised. The pharmaceutical industry has argued for years that clinical trials are expensive, burdensome and time-consuming and therefore hinder the translation of (bio)medical innovation. In the same vein, more recent critical voices have pointed out the mismatch between the highly controlled, experimental nature of randomised placebo-controlled trials and the targeted nature of 'personalised' medicines. They believe that personalised innovations such as regenerative medicine (see Chapter 5), direct-to-consumer genetic testing and other digital health technologies need more flexible, or *real-world* quality and safety evidence instruments to allow for market approval and a swift translation into the clinic.

Echoing this critique, the EMA has undertaken several initiatives in recent years to investigate if – and how – alternative forms of evidence such as real-world evidence could be incorporated within current regulatory science practices. Real-world evidence is understood as "routinely collected data related to a patient's health status or health care delivery from a variety of sources other than traditional clinical trials" (Cave et al 2019, p36). Sources of real-world evidence that are often mentioned in this context are the use of patient-generated (digital health) data or medical information from electronic health records.

Inspired by the US 21st Century Cures Act in 2016, which first introduced the notion of 'alternative evidence', EMA decided to launch the OPTIMAL framework in 2019 to cautiously introduce different forms of real-world evidence within the domain of regulatory science (Cave et al 2019). When it turned out real-world evidence played a pivotal role in providing evidence for effective COVID-19 vaccines, the European Medical Agency decided to expedite its uptake:

> Our vision, anchored in the European Medicines Regulatory Network (EMRN) strategy to 2025, is that by 2025 the use of RWE [real-world evidence] will have been enabled and the value will have been established across the spectrum of regulatory use cases. Delivering this vision will support the development and use of better medicines for patients.
>
> *(Arlett et al 2021, p21)*

Therefore, EMA published several policy documents in recent years to set standards for these forms of evidence, thereby playing a crucial role the infrastructuring of PM in Europe. As already indicated in our previous discussion on the VHT Initiative, efforts to establish the infrastructure for PM in Europe are increasingly linked to a normative assumption that encouraging the creation, collection, management, and storage of medical data will lead to improved healthcare across Europe (European Medicines Agency N.D.). The favourable qualification opinion for Unlearn.AI's TwinRCT solution therefore fits within this datafication reasoning. This infrastructuring of datafication that comes with the EMA's move towards real-world evidence has opened several new spaces of contestation. First, we see a shift in who gets to sit at the table in discussions about EMA policy. Whereas the world of regulatory science-as-we-know-it used to be dominated mainly by large incumbent pharmaceutical firms, this digital move is now giving other players such as Big Tech, digital tech entrepreneurs, engineers, or modellers a seat at the table – players whose vision of the future of biomedical innovations is not necessarily the same as that of Big Pharma. With its move towards real-world evidence, the EMA has also opened a space of contestation around what can be considered 'good evidence' and, indeed, whether regulatory bodies have the right expertise to assess the quality and safety of these complex digital technologies, and determine what is ought to count as 'good' in this new version of regulatory science? With frameworks such as real-world evidence, regulatory bodies also appear to address the regulatory difficulty of digital health by using more digital tools for quality assessment. However, this does not eliminate the question of 'good' digital tools. On the contrary, now that 'quality' is an issue both on the approval side of digital health devices and on the regulatory assessment side the question becomes even more pressing. The question as to what is considered 'good evidence' therefore also opens new questions on who is considered a legitimate expert to develop and assess these real-world evidence criteria (Lievevrouw 2023; Lievevrouw et al 2021).

Secondly, the EMA's attempt to infrastructure PM through real-world evidence frameworks is also opening a space for discussion about the way we understand 'risk'. By quality and safety checking PMs and devices as they are in use, the real-world evidence push is blurring the lines between research and development and actual healthcare practice. The existing framework of quality and safety approvals primarily assumes that pharmaceuticals or medical devices can only be marketed after their quality and safety has been demonstrated, aiming, at least in theory, to reduce the risk of side effects to almost zero (although see Chapter 1). The origins of this risk approach can be traced back to the man-made technological disasters of the twentieth century (e.g., the Thalidomide scandal, Chernobyl, Bhopal), which led to greater reliance by governments on scientific risk assessments as a basis for policy decisions (Abraham 1995; Wynne 2002). Against this backdrop, quality and safety standards have become important tools for governments over the years to limit the risk of harmful health effects from medical products (Demortain 2017).

The 'real-world approach', however, is based on the principle that technological risks can never be brought to zero and should therefore be perceived as matters that can be continuously (digitally) surveilled. With a move towards real-world evidence, the focus of these new EU quality and safety standards shifts from pre-market approval towards post-market surveillance. This move towards post-market surveillance allows for medical (personalised) products – through the use of real-world data – to be brought to market faster, and then – again through the use of real-world data – are to be continuously monitored, allowing (in theory) for speedier 'real-time' response if something goes wrong.

Along this shift to post-market surveillance, EMA's infrastructuring of PM through the development of real-world evidence frameworks blurs the previously clearly separated boundary between medical research and clinical practice. This resonates with prior work by Cambrosio et al (2018) on the rise of molecular and genomic technologies in the field of oncology. They describe a new form of 'experimental care', which is a blending of life-long care with experimental intervention. The question is, how does this shift to 'experimental care' impact individuals in their capacity as both patients and research subjects? (See also Chapter 4). Indeed, this blending – which is inherent to digital health devices – implies that medical data collected through these personalised technologies can be used for multiple different purposes, raising further questions about adequate and appropriate protection for this sensitive data and how to ensure transparency (for patients and the public) about the different ways their health day can and is being used (see Chapter 6). Moreover, the blurring between research and clinic also brings into question issues of accessibility to PM: what about patients or citizens who prefer to refrain from sharing data?

Lastly, this blurring also places a strain on the promise that personalised technologies will enhance patient empowerment. By being used as data-gathering mechanisms for real-world evidence, these PM technologies have become tools for the optimisation of population studies, instead of serving as 'personalised' technologies. In this way, they seem to function as a digital version of biopolitics (Lemke 2001, 2010). Are they re-shaping themselves into a double function of population-monitoring as well as empowerment devices? Is there a distinction between these at all, or is every digital empowerment device, also always a form of population-monitoring (Meyers 2018)?

Conclusion: the politics of infrastructuring PM

This chapter employed the pioneering US 'All of US' Initiative and the EU digital twin initiatives as a lens to examine the infrastructuring of PM as a complex, ongoing, and value-laden process. Rather than viewing infrastructures as static or purely technical systems, this chapter aimed to highlight their socio-technical nature, emerging from and reinforcing particular visions, norms, and power dynamics. Through both case studies, we have shown how infrastructuring efforts therefore always involve value choices, as they are entangled with political, technical, ethical, and social decisions that co-produce (Jasanoff 2004) the development and implementation of PM infrastructures. The chapter showcased this socio-technical infrastructural work in different ways.

A central theme throughout the chapter is that infrastructures for PM do not arise *de novo* but build upon existing installed bases of technical systems, institutional arrangements, and social visions and expectations. This means that infrastructuring is inherently path-dependent and risks reproducing or even exacerbating existing problems. We have shown how the VHT Initiative, for example, is a re-articulation of existing Big Data aspirations, effectively presenting old 'PM' wine in new 'digital twin' bottles. This initiative perpetuates the historical entanglement of PM with Big Data aspirations, continuing the vision of a 'need' for large-scale data aggregation and integration for the advancement of medical research and healthcare delivery. In line with this, the US All of US project illustrates how infrastructuring inclusion is not merely a matter of technical recruitment targets as the project was shaped by deep-rooted structural inequalities, historical mistrust, and the limitations of existing healthcare and research infrastructures.

Moreover, the chapter has shown that PM infrastructurings are performative: they enact particular imaginaries of health, care, and citizenship, often privileging data-intensive, technologically driven solutions over other alternatives. Therefore, infrastructuring is not a neutral or apolitical activity. It rather involves continuous negotiation among diverse actors with competing interests and values, and in doing so opens up new, or re-articulates old spaces of contestation around issues such as inclusion, access, evidence, and risk. This is illustrated in the All of Us initiative, which, despite its efforts to lower barriers to participation through multilingual outreach, flexible consent processes, and community engagement, remains largely focused on enabling research participation rather than ensuring equitable access to the benefits of PM. Its reliance on existing clinical and digital infrastructures therefore risks reproducing at least some of the very exclusions it sought to address. Similarly, the chapter's analysis of the European Medicines Agency's efforts to incorporate digital twins into regulatory frameworks reveals how infrastructuring PM also involves reconfiguring foundational concepts such as 'evidence' and 'risk'. The shift towards real-world evidence and the blurring of boundaries between research and clinical practice raise new critical questions about medical expertise, data protection, health equity, and the meaning of patient empowerment in an increasingly data-driven healthcare landscape.

Processes of infrastructur*ing* and the infrastructures they produce are about the visions, assumptions, and interests of a unique set of supply-side actors: from governments and lawmakers who draw up the policies to bring these infrastructures into being, to the scientists and data collectors who decide which data is useful for which purpose and why some are not. Yet, through all of these decision-making processes, the 'person' at the heart of it all remains, at best, an imagined creature built with datapoints preferred by supply-side actors (as our next chapter reveals), and at worst, subsumed under the conveniently homogenising phrase of *demand-side*. Who is this 'person'? What indeed are their preferences, likes and dislikes? Is the 'person' imagined by the lawmaker the same as the 'person' in scientific research? If these imagined 'persons' are inherently different, whose vision, whose standards and whose infrastructure comes to be instantiated? As we explore these questions in the next chapter, what starts to become clear are the spaces where imaginations and visions converge or diverge, and, perhaps more saliently, the underlying reasons why some infrastructures become the thoroughfares of tomorrow while others disappear.

4

THE PUBLICS OF PERSONALISED MEDICINE

Different personalised medicine initiatives frame their 'publics' in different ways – as patients, consumers, and citizens. Consider the *Citizen Engagement for Personalised Medicine* initiative by the European Union's European Partnership for Personalised Medicine (EP PerMed 2024). At the heart of this initiative lies the notion that this emergent form of medicine – personalised medicine – requires "the formation of new public arenas in which the hopes and responsibilities of [national] citizens become tied more closely to their biology" (Rose and Novas 2005, p26). In contrast to this conceptualisation of the person in personalised medicine is the narrower view of the person as a consumer. When the privately owned genetic-testing enterprise *23andMe* (2024) writes in its marketing material that "your DNA is amazing!" or "welcome to you!" *the person* being addressed is both the 'genetic individual' and the individual-as-consumer. In this framing the 'person' is rendered as "an object of economic, social, and symbolic use" primarily to generate profit (Sharp 2000, p292). Yet another conceptualisation is that of the patient. Defined as "an individual awaiting or under medical care and treatment" (Merriam-Webster 2024), a sociological analysis reveals multiple identities: as an object of study in clinical trials and in the medical classroom; as a subject entitled to some citizen's rights to healthcare, although these rights crucially depend on individual social (age, nationality, geography), economic (affordability for health insurance) and other factors; and as patient-consumers traversing the traditional boundaries of each in untidy and increasingly unprecedented ways (see e.g., Lester 2009). As imaginaries of the *personal* become inextricably intertwined with the *impersonal and standardised,* a useful question to ask is: who this *person* in per-son*alised* medicine is?

In previous chapters we examined the meanings of the *personal* (Chapter 1) and the implications of *personalisation* (Chapter 2). In this chapter, we examine the

DOI: 10.4324/9781003279556-4

question of "who this 'person' in personalised medicine is" through the lens of why and how various actors imagine the *publics* of personalised medicine initiatives. As we will see in this chapter, various actors, including medical professionals, companies developing or selling personalised medicine technologies, and national governments make use of different configurations of the 'person' in personalised medicine. Often their 'publics' are in turn comprised of aggregates of this particular type of 'person'; for example a company selling direct-to-consumer genetic tests might see the 'person' in personalised medicine primarily as a consumer and a set of genetic resources to be collected and turned into assets, and in turn view the relevant 'public' as a (global) market of such consumers waiting to be converted into a pooled set of proprietary data assets. Conversely, a biomedical researcher might see the 'person' in personalised medicine through the lens of biomarker data, and the resulting 'public' as a pool of eligible or ineligible clinical trial participants. People individually and collectively may, to varying degrees, internalise these identities, and act according to the 'scripts' provided by these framings of personhood. Equally, as will be discussed, resistance is not only possible but commonplace. The various identities of the self – whether as a consumer, patient, quantified body, biohacker, biocitizen, or bio-digital citizen – overlap dynamically and are inseparable from each other. A cancer patient may also be self-tracking their health status while consuming genetic testing, claiming their right to cancer care provision by the state and contributing to public engagement initiatives to improve cancer care as a biocitizen. Thus, how a 'person' identifies themselves at any given moment is not only dynamic, based on the needs, interests and aims at any given moment but also overlaps with multiple identities. A more pragmatic approach to understanding the 'person of personalised medicine' is to investigate how various identities – research subject, research object, consumer, patient, quantified self, biohacker, citizen, and so on – are imagined.

Imagining publics

While a definition of 'publics' is elusive, most agree on its basic characteristics. The first relates to the identity of publics: despite publics being transient and dynamic, they are a "specifiable and discernible entity that is inextricable from its conditions of origin" (Dewey 1927 in Di Salvo 2009, p49). Following from this, the second characteristic relates to how publics form, based on "indirect, extensive, enduring, and serious consequences of conjoint and interacting behaviour" around a specific context or issue (Dewey 1927, p126). The third relates to why publics form and Dewey's reflection on this suggests consequentialist motivations in the sense that publics form "with a common interest in controlling [the] consequences [of the context or issue in question]" (Dewey, 1927, p126). As such, Dewey's conceptualisation of publics is an expansive one; he not only imagined a plurality of such entities co-forming and co-existing but also that they may be formed "for good or evil" aims (Dewey 1927, p35 in Di Salvo 2009, p50). The key elements are that publics exist in relation to something other than merely themselves, and that they are purposeful. Public spheres across myriad emerging technologies today largely reflect this expansive notion. From data-driven and/or AI-enabled technologies such as personalised medicine, facial recognition to social media, vaccines, or green technologies, the public spheres of each are populated by a plurality and diversity of publics, with *good* or *bad* motivations from supporting conspiracy theories, technology-scepticism, private vested interests to improving access to public goods, better oversight, social justice, and trade promotion.

In contrast, stakeholder engagement initiatives, whether by the state, civil society, or industry groups, typically conceptualise a much narrower notion of *publics* as 'citizens' based on the rights and responsibilities of national citizenship (discussed below). At the same time, 'citizens' are neither homogenous nor an uncomplex imaginary. For instance, the institutionalisation of public engagement (consultation) as part of the formal processes of policymaking or legitimising discourse, especially in technology development, has led to the emergence of divergent and dynamic 'imaginaries' of publics (Welsh and Wynne 2013). Likewise, the traditional perception of 'citizens' by state actors as uncritical, unreflexive passive recipients of public services have expanded as diverse – and often critical – publics have emerged in response to perceived gaps in the state provisioning and oversight of personalised medicine. At the same time, imaginaries of the self as the 'whole person' as a social or emotional being are increasingly destabilised by the evolving imperatives of the quantified 'person' defined primarily in terms of biological and digital data (Morrison and Kelly 2021). Yet, even as the 'quantified self' has drawn on narratives of empowerment and agency to evolve into sub-cultural identities and consumerist movements, an increasing number of people have kept their distance, viewing "self-tracking tools as part of a culture of surveillance" as disempowering and undesirable (Sharon 2017, p99).

Thus, the answer to the question we asked earlier "who are the publics?" appears to lie in, and vary with, how different actors imagine their publics, shaped largely by their vision for shaping technology development and implementation. As noted in Chapter 1, developers of personalised medicine technologies must anticipate the roles and capacities of the people with whom the technology is intended to interact. Moreover, the narratives of personalised medicine are tailored to appeal to different audiences. Thus, the users and other publics of personalised medicine are actively constructed and imagined by different groups in different ways. A more pragmatic approach is thus to ask, 'how are publics imagined?' and in the next section, we investigate this question through the lens of the three key actors – science, society, and state.

Science, biomarkers, and patients: research subjects or research objects?

For scientists and researchers engaged with various strands of personalised medicine research including clinical trials, *patients* are perceived to represent the imagined public of PM. The bulk of the literature on clinical trials for personalised medicine imagines *patients* as entities characterised by their biomarkers. The word choice of 'entities' to describe *patients*, which some readers may find curious or even offensive, argues for the decontextualisaion of the research subject from their social milieu. A key player in our understanding here is the term *biomarker* – short for biological markers – and defined as "a characteristic that is objectively measured and evaluated as an indicator of normal biological processes, pathogenic processes, or pharmacologic responses to a therapeutic intervention", which may be diagnostic, prognostic, or predictive (Biomarkers Definition Working Group 2001). Genetic and genomic data is one form of biomarker but there are many others. Before a clinical trial for personalised medicine can begin, the commonest form being the 'enrichment trial', biomarker profiles of potential patients are validated (or analysed) (Superchi et al 2022, p1). Only patients with the biomarker of interest to the study (i.e., biomarker-positive patients) are accepted for the trial and "randomly assigned to the targeted or control arms" (Superchi et al 2022, p1), while those without the biomarker of interest (i.e., biomarker-negative patients) are rejected from participation in the trial. The *public* for research(ers) in personalised medicine is characterised by their biomarker profiles, driven by the hope of emulating the success of a few biomarkers; namely, *Herceptin* for HER2 (human epidermal growth factor receptor 2)-positive breast cancer patients and *imatinib mesylate* for chronic myeloid leukaemia (Lawler and Sullivan 2015, p2). Yet, the benefits and implications of biomarker-driven approaches for patients vary considerably based on genetic heterogeneity, demographics, geography, and socioeconomic determinants.

A primary implication of patient heterogeneity can be seen in the unevenness and uncertainties of clinical outcomes. Janiaud et al (2019) observed that

> the diversity in biomarkers combined with the unique evolution of malignant tumours (i.e., tumour growth and spread may be accompanied by changes in the biomarker profile) challenge the ability of traditional cancer trials to test targeted therapies with enough statistical power due to high inter- and intra-patient heterogeneity.
>
> *(p21)*

Furthermore, this dynamic heterogeneity not only "make[s] it difficult to acquire evidence on the benefit of novel therapeutics, but also on the validity and clinical use of biomarkers, creating a large gap between biomarker discoveries and their clinical translation" (Janiaud et al 2019, p21).

A fundamental, and to an extent ontological, question here is whether the so-called biomarker-positive or -negative *patients* are 'patients' in any meaningful way since:

> [biomarkers] may but do not necessarily correlate with a patient's experience and sense of wellbeing, and it is easy to imagine measurable biological

> characteristics that do not correspond to patients' clinical state, or whose variations are undetectable and without effect on health. It is also even easier to imagine measurable biological characteristics whose variance among populations is so great as to render them all but useless as reliable predictors of disease or its absence.
>
> *(Strimbu and Tavel 2010, p2)*

Despite these uncertainties and unevenness in 'correlating' biomarkers to standard clinical endpoints (such as diagnosing and curing disease, and improving wellbeing), biomarkers have profound implications for patient's lived experiences. These issues of correlation and consequence are present when making (or not) a diagnosis, as discussed in relation to genetic and genomic data in Chapter 2, and equally, though in subtly different ways, manifest in relation to trial access and treatment pathways.

On the one hand, biomarker-positive (or negative) *patients* in clinical trials are little more than research subjects, reduced to a set of qualifying biomarker validation criteria based on the inclusion or exclusion criteria of the clinical trial. This, it is reasonable to argue, is neither new nor unusual but simply the language of clinical trials or any scientific research for that matter. Clinical practice and clinical trials represent two parallel worlds guided by different sets of aims and outcomes. As Strimbu and Tavel (2010, p2) observe:

> The goal of clinical practice is to improve morbidity and mortality, [but] not to change quantifiable features of patients' innate biochemistry, for instance, with no outward clinical effect. Similarly, patients seek treatment for their diseases, not for the numerical measures that frequently but not perfectly correlate with their illnesses.

Yet, these two worlds of research and practice are increasingly colliding in unprecedented and unexpected ways in biomarker-driven PM studies, questioning assumptions grounded in traditional research-practice boundaries, as demarcation lines – between clinical endpoints and clinical research; between research subjects and research objects – become increasingly blurred (Cambrosio et al 2024; Polk et al 2023). A germane example is a fieldwork note (among many) by Cambrosio and colleagues (2024, p507) produced during their qualitative study of the interrelationships between patients, clinical staff, and researchers at the New York-based Memorial Sloan Kettering Cancer Center's Early Drug Development Service. Cambrosio and colleagues observe how two oncologists from differing specialisations set up:

> a 'pipeline' of these trials, whereby patients expressing the biomarker would progress through available studies in a predetermined sequence, based on an emerging hypothesis about how some agents may, in addition to their primary

> therapeutic effects, serve as primers of the immune system for response to subsequent agents [...] inspired by the observation [made] in previous trials [...] with the possibility of greater clinical benefit if the hypothesis is correct, while potentially generating insights for further biological investigation.
>
> *(Cambrosio et al 2024, p507)*

This increasingly blurred research subject-object boundaries, however, is not only limited to the clinician's perspective but also reflects the similarly blurred lived experiences of affected patients as those who joined the 'pipeline' earlier were expected to show a better response to treatment. With the result that "even if there are standard [treatment] options available [clinicians] sometimes recommended to patients that perhaps [they] should consider [a]particular clinical trial" (Polk et al 2023, p5). Implicit here are the contingent multi-layered complexities of advancing the field of biomarker-driven *precision oncology*. As the note shows, realising the scientific vision of probabilistic quantification of disease depends increasingly on research(ers) ability to negotiate and integrate with the patient-centred world of clinical practice or what McWhinney (1989, p876) has called "the patient's world, [where the physician tries] to see the illness through the patient's eyes".[1]

Yet, the slow pace of translating biomarker-driven approaches from bench to bedside suggests that research-practice intersections, especially at scale, have been rare, and largely limited to settings where such interactions were already in place such as in large university (teaching) hospitals. In turn, this has contributed to poor consideration of "clinical needs [as] a starting point for the development of biomarkers" and considered by many to be symptomatic of systemic weaknesses in the biomarker development 'pipeline' (Ioannidis and Bossuyt 2017, p963). As a result, the publics imagined by research(ers) of biomarker-driven approaches remain stubbornly limited to the *patient as a research subject* – detached and decontextualised from the patient's lived experience of the disease. The body of scientific literature, especially those related to clinical trials, evidences this (discussed later). In turn, this raises questions about the extent to which missed attention to the patient's personal and clinical needs will eventually play out in terms of social (clinical, patient) acceptability of "numerical measures that frequently but not perfectly correlate with illnesses" (Strimbu and Tavel 2010, p2).

A related issue is the broader social acceptability implications of biomarker-driven approaches to personalised treatment. Of particular concern is the exclusion of certain subpopulations from biomarker-driven studies based on quantified measurements, such as biomarker-negative individuals. Exclusion and inclusion criteria are an integral part of research design and that biomarker-driven approaches should follow these design protocols is accepted and expected. The issue is that treatments developed through biomarker-driven studies will mostly benefit the subgroups studied, while those excluded from studies are unlikely to benefit.

This is because the logic of personalised medicine works by inverting the traditional drug discovery approach of finding a treatment first before trialling it on patients. Instead, the "the clinical utility of a biomarker (in its role as the companion diagnostic for a specific new therapy) is defined by its ability to reliably identify a patient subgroup that benefits from the new therapy" (Freidlin and Korn 2014, p81). Since biomarker-driven 'personalised' approaches to treatments produce a "heterogeneity of treatment effects" the success of the approach lies in "develop[ing] biomarkers to identify patients who could benefit from new treatments" (Freidlin and Korn 2014, p81). For instance, most of the emerging "new anticancer treatments [which] are molecular targeted agents [that] only benefit a subgroup of patients within a histologically defined cancer" (Freidlin and Korn 2014, p81). One such treatment is the *Cetuximab*, an anti-epidermal growth factor receptor (EGFR) monoclonal antibody for administration in addition to first-line chemotherapy treatment of patients with EGFR-positive metastatic colorectal cancer (mCRC). A large-scale clinical study to evaluate *Cetuximab's* effectiveness found that it does "reduce the risk of progression of mCRC when used as the first-line treatment" (Van Cutsem et al 2009, p1416). However, since "this benefit is seen mainly in patients with wild-type–KRAS tumours" (Van Cutsem et al 2009, p1416), researchers have argued that 'overall-effect' trials including entire subpopulations "could have impaired …the detection of the benefit of Cetuximab in the KRAS wild-type subgroup" (Freidlin and Korn 2014, p81). Note that 'wild type' is a term used by geneticists to refer to the most common form of a gene variant found in a given population. It is typically considered to be the normal or baseline version of a gene against which other versions are identified as variant mutations. In the above examples KRAS is a gene which helps to regulate cell growth and division and can therefore lead to tumour formation (abnormal cell growth) if it develops a harmful mutation.

The key point here is that researchers argue conducting trials on biomarker-positive subgroups (e.g., with KRAS wild-type biomarker in the above cases) produces a more robust evaluation of treatment efficacy (clinical utility) for that specific subgroup. This suggests that efficacy findings would have been less robust had the trials been conducted on the entire subpopulation (including biomarker-negative subgroups) to measure the average treatment effect. Thus, clinical literature widely recommends 'subgroup-specific approaches' for more effective treatment discovery, particularly recommending the use of 'enrichment trials' *enriched* with smaller biomarker-positive subgroups (instead of randomised overall-type trials) as most efficient in terms of delivering robust clinical evidence of *treatment efficacy* (Freidlin and Korn 2014; Graf et al 2015; Krisam and Kieser 2014, 2015; Mehta et al 2014) as well as *cost-effectiveness* (Lawler and Sullivan 2015; McShane et al 2023; see "prognostic enrichment" in Cheng et al 2020).

However, such 'subgroup-specific approaches' have profound implications for the patient's lived experience of treatment and for society where the implications of stratifying, excluding, and including patients using numerical tools are substantive. While a reflection on or study of these implications is largely missing across the clinical literature, a growing body of social science scholarship explore the implicit clinical uncertainties (Hauge 2024). In particular, sociological analyses focus on understanding the wide 'spectrum' rather than 'binary' nature of biomarker 'actionability' (Tarantino et al 2021), which is defined as the "aim to generate predictive relationships between genetic information and drug therapies" (Nelson et al 2013, p405). Instead, many scholars interested in the societal aspects argue that "making genetic mutation data actionable depends on the constraints posed by related socio-technical systems – and several such considerations are involved when assessing alternative courses of action" (Nelson et al 2013, p14). These considerations range from "the regulatory status of [...] mutations and drugs, the availability of testing and treatments within health care systems, and the geographical location and design of clinical trials for drugs still under development" (Nelson et al 2013, p14; see also Tempini and Leonelli 2021, p2). Considerations of patients' lived experience are also salient here, for example, among parents of children with disabilities (Stivers and Timmermans 2017) and that of clinical actors entrusted with their care (Rabeharisoa and Bourret 2009).

A further issue is the plight of biomarker-negative patients; how clinical outcomes can be less positive for those who have other forms of the disease, and indeed for the clinicians who are treating them. This was illustrated in Chapter 1 through the case of *trastuzumab* (Herceptin), a breast cancer drug linked to high levels of a particular cell surface receptor as a biomarker. *Trastuzumab* has little benefit for breast cancer patients who do not have high levels of HER2, but their condition is no less serious despite not gaining any new therapies. What is further problematic from a societal perspective is that once a targeted medicine receives marketing approval, firms have relatively little incentive to produce robust evidence of its utility (or not) in other patient populations (Chapter 1). For instance, after *trastuzumab* was approved for women with HER2 positive breast cancers in 1998, it took a further 20 years of work to accumulate enough evidence that women with HER2 negative cancers did not receive any significant benefit (Kimmelman and Tannock 2018).

Society and agency: of consumers, patients, and resisters

An interrogation of how society imagines its relationship with emerging science and technology is inevitably also an interrogation of agency and self-determination against the "[governing] techniques which assure coercion and processes through which the self is constructed or modified by himself" (Foucault 1993, p203–204). In emerging technological areas like personalised medicine, "governing techniques" [or what we might call governance infrastructures] tend to be in their earliest developmental phases and relatively flexible earlier in the process but becoming increasingly inflexible over time as development advances (Collingridge 1980, p11). As a result, the extent to which publics have agency in (not) choosing to *use* a certain technology vary substantially based on where the technology is along its developmental trajectory. In turn, this has profound implications for how publics imagine their relationship with an emerging (personalised medicine) technology in terms of responsibilisation and individualisation of healthcare – whether as consumers, patients, or resisters.

Consumers

Defined as "a person who buys goods or services for their own use" (Cambridge Dictionary 2024), *the consumer* and the imaginary of publics as 'consumers' is inextricably intertwined with the multi-layered and contingent complexities of consumer choice. However, how consumers make rational choices (for a discussion of 'consumer choice theory' – see Thaler 1980) between a variety of goods and services depends largely on 'usable' knowledge of the product (Ravetz 1987). The latter is based on 'available' information but crucially taking into account the human cognitive limitations to processing the vast information available today or what is known as 'bounded rationality' (see e.g. Dequech 2001; Simon 1997). In the case of emerging science and technology such as personalised medicine, consumer access to available information and the boundedness conditions underlying how much of this is usable for decision-making has implications for how publics understand and accept emerging scientific knowledge (for a discussion of the 'public understanding of science' see Bauer 2009; Brossard and Lewenstein 2009; for a discussion on the social acceptability of the emerging science and technology and the framing concept of 'responsible' innovation see Stilgoe et al 2013).

At the same time, autonomy of consumer choice in health and medicine is also about the individual consumer responsibility for their own health decisions, bringing to the forefront issues of individualisation of responsibility which accompany the personalisation of health. Self-tracking applications (apps) and wearable devices (wearables) measuring anything from steps, heartbeats, blood sugar, menstruation cycles and sleeping patterns to moods have shifted "the paradigm of the old thinking 'My health is the responsibility of my physician', [to] the new thinking that 'My health is my responsibility, and I have the tools to manage it'" (Swan 2012, p108). This has rendered the individual consumer of health goods and services as what Tutton and Prainsack call the 'enterprising self'

> who is addressed through a discourse of democratisation and empowerment, and who has the right to information as a value in itself [...] this participant is engaged in a consumer transaction by which she both purchases and provides information about herself.
>
> *(2011, p1090)*

On the one hand, the easy availability of direct-to-consumer health goods like self-tracking tools have bolstered various policy narratives responsibilising the 'self' for good health by leading healthy lifestyles. For instance, the UK National Health Service's "Better Health – More ways to kick-start *your heath*" (emphasis added) campaign responsibilises the individual for leading a healthy lifestyle and provides six different self-tracking tools (apps) on its website to achieve this as below:

> More ways to kickstart your health
>
> Healthy changes start with little changes. Whether you want to lose weight, drink less alcohol, get active or quit smoking, you have access to lots of free tools and support through Better Health. You can also find simple ways to lift your mood with Every Mind Matters.
>
> There has never been a better time to kickstart your health. Let's do this!
>
> - NHS Food Scanner app – Start finding healthier swaps today!
> - NHS Weight Loss Plan – A 12-week plan to help you lose weight. Couch to 5K app – A running app for absolute beginners.
> - Active 10 app – Track and build up your daily walks–start with 10 minutes every day!
> - Drink Free Days app – For the days you do not want to drink alcohol.
> - NHS Quit Smoking app – Daily support to help you quit smoking and start breathing easier.
>
> *(NHS N.D.)*

In turn, these policy narratives have gained currency as a strategy for reducing costs and activities among public health organisations that are held 'responsible' for disease prevention and provisioning public health (Hutchison and Holdsworth 2021).

On the other hand, the emergence of the 'quantified self' as a self-optimising consumer of health and lifestyle-centred goods and services has enabled the construction of novel "subcultural identities [emblematic] of the expressive or stylistic dimensions of everyday life" (Michael 1998, p316). Consider the 'quantified self' communities of "individual[s] engaged in the self-tracking of any kind of biological, physical, behavioural, or environmental information" (Swan 2013, p85). From an imagined public of isolated consumers, each self-quantifying using various metrics, electronic, and digital tools, the notion has evolved into 'communities' integrating all these individual data into a communal or 'group data', which not only allows for comparisons between each other but also collaborations within the 'quantified' communities (Swan 2013). Viewed this way, the consumer imaginary of self-tracking, self-optimising technologies is "no longer seen to be a matter of [publics] consuming things simply because these enable the accomplishment of certain material ends or the performance of certain practical functions" but adding layers of complexities (in the form of social relations and interactions) to emerging identities and communities leading to the evolution of novel subcultures (Michael 1998, p316).

Increasingly, however, these emerging subcultures of consumption are not only shaping how scientific knowledge is consumed (Michael 1998, p317) but also how it is produced. Consider for example, the 'biohacking' community. The idea of 'biohacking' builds on self-tracking cultures and the notion of the 'quantified self' to control and improve the biology of the self through "a distinct though overlapping mode of contemporary techno-asceticism [in the sense of self-improvement] with its own set of norms and frameworks for bodily self-use ... including its simultaneous alignment with alternative health cultures" (Lindfors 2024, p83). Biohacking is thus at once about striving towards the idealised 'natural' self as it is necessarily about using the artificial, digitised and datafied means to attain these ends. In this sense, biohackers are just another emerging typology of the self-imagined publics of personalised medicine, but one that increasingly challenges the claims to exclusive legitimacy of credentialed scientific expertise. Consider Dave Asprey, author of two successful biohacking 'guidebooks' – *The Bulletproof Diet* and *Head Strong*. Asprey is neither a clinician nor a scientist but according to the Amazon page selling his book:

> a Silicon Valley entrepreneur [who] has worked with world-renowned doctors and scientists to uncover the latest, most innovative methods for making humans perform better – a process known as 'biohacking'.
>
> *(Asprey 2017)*

Asprey's recommended "[two-week program of] simple lifestyle modifications (or 'hacks') ... to take [publics'] mental performance to the next level" include actions such as:

> which foods to eat and which ones to avoid, how to incorporate the right kinds of physical activity into your day, a detox protocol for your home and body; meditation and breathing for performance, recommended brain-boosting supplements; and how to adjust the lighting in your home and workspace to give your brain the quality light it thrives on.
>
> *(Asprey 2017)*

On the face of it, Asprey's recommended actions are neither novel nor markedly transformative. Except perhaps that they build on the evolving subcultural identities of the 'quantified self' to argue for what might be loosely described as a countercultural movement away from the gold standard of scientific knowledge. Instead, it pushes biomedical knowledge production towards a more socially constructed direction aligned with 'nature', "balancing the 'masculine' reason of its technoscientific leanings with a 'feminine' intuition, embodied knowledge and a sensory cosmology drawn from alternative health cultures" (Lindfors 2024, p84). Yet, it is not always the transformative ideology of the Biohackers that draws publics to the 'Quantified Self' movements. Rather, it might just be the basal human desire for 'community' – to be part of "a social life of sharing" the self – where the awkwardness many associate with socialising is overcome by the simple fact that even if "you might not always have something to say, …you always have a number to report" (Gary Wolf, co-founder of the Quantified Self movement in Wolf 2010). Viewed this way, the imaginary of publics as 'consumers' is increasingly inextricably intertwined not only with the multi-layered complexities of consumer choice, but also increasingly tied up with individual preferences (choices) for shaping the knowledge itself (of self-tracking tool in this instance) in novel and unprecedented ways as a pre-condition for 'consuming' it. The result is a process of stretching, expanding and re-interpreting what counts as 'usable' knowledge of self-tracking tools by individualising and re-inventing its consumption (usability, use) in interaction with the agency of the self, and human body.

Patients

At the same time, the lived realities of disease and illness as a patient (or as a close family or friend of a patient) changes, at times irrevocably, the interrelationships between the self, autonomy to choose, and the desperation to access novel treatments and therapies that offer relief or cure from suffering and death. This is especially the case for terminal conditions or debilitating diseases (such as cancer and multiple sclerosis) where there were no safe or effective treatments before. In the language of demand and supply, the lived realities of disease often create an unchangeable (inelastic) demand for its treatment independent of the conditions of its supply including its price at the point of care. The latter issue of pricing (or reimbursement) is highly significant and contentious in emerging personalised medicine, which is typically prohibitively costly, and access for the majority is inevitably tied to affordability considerations. For instance, a single treatment of Kymriah (tisagenlecleucel), a cell therapy (see Chapter 5) for treating Acute lymphoblastic leukaemia (ALL) in children and young adults' costs over US$612,000 or an estimated £282,000 per patient in the UK (Blood Cancer-UK 2018).

Likewise, Yescarta (axicabtagene ciloleucel), a one-time treatment for B-cell lymphoma costs US$485,021 per patient. Thus, for the vast majority of those suffering from diseases and/or conditions for which personalised therapeutics are available but only accessible at the mercy of the insurer's reimbursement calculus or health technology assessment (see Chapter 5 for more discussions of how rationing practices introduce further stratification of access to personalised medicines), the question of agency or consumer 'choice' does not arise. For instance, 800 people each year in the UK are diagnosed with the lethal blood cancer B-cell acute lymphoblastic leukaemia (B-cell ALL). However, it was estimated that only 40 children and young adults across England and Wales would be eligible for free treatment with the cell therapy Kymriah based on cost-benefit assessments made by the UK national medicines commissioner The National Institute for Health and Care Excellence (NICE) (Pinches 2024). This is the lived reality of patienthood in emerging personalised medicine, where individuals are far from being *consumers* exercising their freedom to (not) choose their own treatment pathways. Rather, as the example of Kymriah shows, the vast majority are desperate *patients* with little, if any, agency over their own healthcare decisions including the choice of living over dying. As one young patient from Liverpool, who received Kymriah through early access to innovative available scheme under the UK NHS' Cancer Drugs Fund[2] put it:

> Without this drug, I faced very limited options, and had a relatively poor prognosis, and would have otherwise engaged in palliative care conversations.
> *('Sophie' quoted in Pinches 2024 [online])*

In many ways, this imaginary of patienthood in personalised medicine defined by limited (if any) autonomy over the fate of the self and at the mercy of structural pressures related to affordability and accessibility is in stark contrast to the imaginary of the consumer especially the 'Quantified Self' or biohacking movements. At the same time, each of these different identities highlights the inevitability of Foucauldian biopolitical governance and surveillance albeit via different pathways; the quantified-self subjugated to the biopolitics of datafied, systemised quantification of the body and the patient subjugated to the datafied, systematised 'scarcity' of public health provision.

Resisters

Beyond consumers and patients is a third imaginary of publics comprised of those hesitant and sceptical about or resistant to the datafication, responsibilisation and tracking of the self. For some, resistance to imperatives of self-responsibilisation for health and well-being is simply a matter of lacking the resources, whether in terms of money, time, or capacity, to adopt the recommended 'healthier lifestyle choices'. Where responsibility is framed in terms of consumer choice, more expensive 'healthier' options may simply be unaffordable. Similarly, injunctions to 'get more exercise' are often not a viable option for people who lack access to safe, accessible outdoor spaces. Others may resist or reject the moral framing of 'choice' offered by predictive, data driven technologies. Susan Kelly (2009) has studied the reproductive choices of parents of children with serious genetic conditions in the United States. Due to already having one child with a genetic condition, these parents are considered at 'high risk' of having future children with genetic diseases and are typically recommended to undergo pre-implantation genetic screening of the embryo for any future pregnancies, with a view to having the choice to abort pregnancies judged likely to result in an affected child. However, many parents choose to have no more children, as this avoids having to make the choices of whether to reject genetic screening, risking having a second affected child, or accepting embryo screening and risk having to decide whether or not to undergo an abortion. As Kelly notes, they 'choose not to choose'. By doing so they resist the dominant (medical) framing of genetic testing as enabling parents to make the choice to have healthy children. This resistance is, as Kelly argues, an active decision rather than a passive one: "Choosing not to choose was an active response to dilemmas raised by social and technical practices of reproductive genetics, experiences of childhood impairment, and parents' views of risk, responsibility and self" (Kelly 2009, p93).

Another reason for resistance to quantification and self-monitoring is resistance to perceptions of overt and covert biomedical surveillance inherent in these technologies and its implications for the biopolitical governance of the self and publics (Foucault 1997). Sharon (2017) has argued that while many see self-tracking as empowering in that it brings power over the medical body back to the self, 'resisters' hold a somewhat opposite view. For these resisters,

> self-tracking tools as part of a culture of surveillance implies that far from empowering individuals to be more in control, self-tracking for health is disempowering, insofar as it invites an increased control of others–health–promoters, friends and followers, and even the internalized health promoter of one's own super ego – over oneself.
>
> *(Sharon 2017, p99)*

These concerns are increasingly emphasised in the fast-growing use of self-tracking data by insurance providers for risk-assessment purposes primarily with the aim of 'personalising risk' (McFall 2019). This has profound implications for public health. McFall (2019, p54) has argued that personalising the price of health and other insurance products based on individuated risk assessments drawn from self-tracking data is also to "simultaneously personalize access to care". Since this suggests that access to care is now differentiated based on individual lifestyle and behavioural choices, well beyond traditional risk factors like age and health status, it invariably raises profound questions about privacy and biopolitical surveillance. Consider Christophersen and colleagues' (2015) study of how corporate 'wellness programs' in US-based self-insured organisations shape the use of wearable health-tracking devices. Through the lens of policies aimed at reducing health-insurance costs, Christophersen et al (2015) reveal how self-tracking tools are increasingly used by companies to 'enforce' behavioural change among employees, especially how they use financial incentives to encourage employee use of tracking devices to record health targets (Goldberg 2012; Satariano 2014) and disincentives (fines) for those who refuse to participate[3] (Christophersen et al 2015).

Whether this latter group who refuse or resist participation in self-tracking or biohacking count as publics of personalised medicine is, for us, an academic question that provides future research opportunities. Our aim in this section is to present a 'full picture' of the publics of personalised medicine from the perspective of 'society' regardless of whether these publics are the affected or the disaffected. An overriding reason is also the fact that the numbers in this group (of resisters) are not inconsequential. For instance, an online Statista survey of 2,301 adult US-residents conducted between

October 2017 and January 2018 found that 20% of respondents were unwilling to wear technology that measures and tracks (Statista 2025). Likewise, a recent survey conducted online on a nationally representative sample of 1,181 adults in the US found "a sizeable third (32%) of respondents chose the category 'Not applicable – I have never tracked my health using a device or app'" (Nguyen 2024). While better evidence is required to substantiate claims that 'sceptics' of self-tracking are on the rise, that substantial number of people who refuse or resist participation should give pause to accounts of the dominance or inevitability of PM.

On the one hand, this 'resistance' raises questions and public concern about biopolitical governance, from concerns about reducing health and wellbeing to measurable numbers, oftentimes to arrive at an economistic value (Datta Burton 2022) to concerns about the encroaching normalisation of biopolitical surveillance and monitoring in our lives (Foucault 1975). Recent data shows this is increasingly the concern for a growing number. For instance, an online survey of 16- to 18-year-old school students in the United Kingdom found that "[a]lmost half (46%) of the teens [did] not think that self-tracking tools should be used in schools" (Freeman and Neff 2023, p3055–3056). Key concerns were about "losing control of their self-tracked data and want[ing] to maintain a sense of *agency* over their choice of whether to self-track or not" and *surveillance* "that self-tracking could introduce unwanted pressure to perform if their physical activity is quantified" (Freeman and Neff 2023, p3055–3056; emphasis added). In another mixed method survey (including interviews) to understand why publics reject self-tracking apps, findings across the 67 respondents revealed the top reasons were: 'digital unfamiliarity' with self-tracking technologies, general 'rejection of technologisation' as a means of knowing the self, 'negative effects [on the self] such as stress and culpability', and perceptions of 'self-quantification as a constraint' based on rejection of "dependen[cies] on these types of devices [with] some express[ing] hesitations towards the storage and use of their data" (Hargis and Régnier 2018, p1–2).

In many ways, these issues are symptomatic of increasing public mistrust of scientific evidence in general (Datta 2020) and digital tools in particular especially those intended for tracking (Hargis and Régnier 2018, p1–2). It is now a common challenge of advancing digitalisation, building on widespread perceptions of new and oftentimes unknown forms of internet-mediated threats to agency, autonomy, and privacy especially after several high profile revelations of contentious large-scale surveillance, such as Edward Snowden's revelations of the US state's surveillance of citizens in 2013 (Macaskill and Dance 2013), and Frances Haugen's revelation of Facebook's surveillance of its users and its disregard for online harm (Milmo 2021). While the extent to which these issues will impact the publics of personalised medicine – where researcher's access to and use of personal health data remains central to the project – not only depend on publics' trust in how their data is handled but also how oversight processes are able to implement and enforce the checks and balances of data-handling needed to earn and build that trust (this will be discussed in the context of data protection in Chapter 6).

The role of the state: imagining 'good' citizens and citizenship

For state actors, all manner of publics and technology stakeholders within national borders typically get clubbed together under the umbrella term 'citizens'. This is expected and underscored by the relationship between the state and its polity conferring the rights and responsibilities of national citizenship. The issue is that 'citizens' are a highly heterogeneous group and in the case of personalised medicine, differentiated broadly by how their function is imagined by the state, with the commonest being as:

a **contributors,** contributing to the societally aligned shaping of technology development and implementation through participation in various public engagement and other consultative processes, and
b **beneficiaries** of the state provision of public health services as well as effective oversight of health goods and services.

Citizens as contributors to the shaping of technology development

The imaginary of citizen-publics in the role of contributors to technology development and implementation conceives of 'citizens' in a narrower sense of not only being 'good' citizens of good social standing but also 'interested' in delivering or improving public goods (Rose 1999). The defining characteristics of 'good' and 'interested' to imagine the citizen is salient here. For how these words are interpreted and thereafter used to frame narratives of citizenship play a significant role in shaping technology development and implementation in general and particularly in the case of personalised medicine.

Who or what is this 'good' citizen? While a definitive answer is elusive across the body of Science and Technology Studies (STS) scholarship, what emerges across the range of stakeholder initiatives now used by the state, civil society, or industry groups to seek citizen contributions are the frames of "engage[ment] by competent citizens" (Dryzek 2000, p1) or 'representative participants' (Gutmann and Thompson 1996) to describe 'good' citizenship. Consider the 'Personalised Medicine for the European Citizen: Towards more precise medicine for the diagnosis, treatment and prevention of disease (iPM)' initiative by the European Science Foundation (2012). In describing the 'European Citizen', the initiative notes the below:

> *Data shared by patients* have already been used effectively for research purposes and it is apparent that *this sort of citizen-led collaboration* can serve to accelerate clinical research. …Furthermore, ensuring that citizens are able to play an active role in their own healthcare and supporting the *wellbeing of others in their communities* is an important aspect of promoting future participatory healthcare.
>
> *(European Science Foundation 2012, pxiv; emphasis added).*

Likewise, the US National Institute of Health's All of Us Program (see also Chapter 3) evokes a similar communitarian ethos to take forward its aim for "accelerating research advances and precision medicine", writing that:

> Come aboard the *All of Us* Journey, ...to learn how *you can help shape the future of health for yourself, your family, your community, and generations to come.*
>
> *(All of US 2023, emphasis added)*

Implicit in these descriptions is the normative commitment of a 'good' citizen to various community-centred actions to deliver common goods from sharing data to working with others in accelerating research with and for the wellbeing of others. This evokes the imaginary of what Tutton and Prainsack's (2011, p1090) has called the 'altruistic self' "who is addressed through a discourse of communitarianism, and who donates their biomedical data freely, giving of themselves with no expectation of anything in return" (Tutton and Prainsack 2011, p1090).

At the same time, the conceptualisation of the 'citizen' is not merely about the individual or the community. Rather it is emblematic of the "formation of new public arenas in which the hopes and responsibilities of citizens become tied more closely to their biology" (Rose and Novas 2005, p26). As the European Science Foundation's (2012, p17), Personalised Medicine for the European Citizen. Towards more precise medicine for the diagnosis, treatment and prevention of disease (iPM) initiative notes:

> Patients who are willing to participate fully can hope to receive not only tailored treatment once diseases have developed, therefore, but also tailored prevention strategies based on a *continuously updated biological profile*. Despite the assertion that medicine has always been personalised, it is clear that in many areas citizens have not felt that they are fully in control of the decisions made about their wellbeing. Personalised medicine could provide the means for citizens to exert more control over their health without having to rely directly on professional healthcare. [...] *This is a potentially empowering step for European citizens.*
>
> *(emphasis added)*

This entanglement of citizenship with personalised medicine here is undoubtedly tied to agency and empowerment of the individual (see e.g., Tutton and Prainsack's [2011] 'enterprising self' discussed earlier). At the same time, it is about the incremental divestment of state responsibility away from delivering public health provision towards individualisation of responsibility. Viewed this way, the imaginary of the 'good citizen' is intrinsically tied to the ways their 'goodness' vis-a-vis community-centred actions of (data) sharing can help them to become 'empowered citizens', while shifting away from the governmentality of public health provision as a *citizen's right* to *a citizen's responsibility*. It is against this backdrop of emerging governmentality, shifting state responsibility away from citizens' health to (data) extractivism, that the authors of the European Science Foundation's (2012, p40–41) report caution that:

> However, [empowerment of the European citizen] will require a genuine devolution of power and agency to the citizen. Token measures used ostensibly to empower citizens will not be effective if the central aim is merely to encourage them to give up data and intellectual property rights in order that they can be used and exploited by others. It should also be remembered, however, that *participation will inevitably be variable* and some groups will need to *delegate responsibility for their care back to the healthcare profession.*
>
> *(emphasis added)*

Following from this, and specifically given the unevenness of participation (partly acknowledged in the comment above and fleshed out in our discussion of PM 'resisters' above), a relevant question is who or what is this 'interested' citizen participating in technology development and implementation? Nicolas Rose (1999) has argued that building this 'competent citizenry' rarely, if ever, happens in a void. Rather, it is *manufactured* by professionals who Rose calls "experts of community [formation]" using "a whole array of little devices and techniques ... invented to make communities real" (Rose 1999, p189–190). With advancing entrenchment of public (stakeholder) engagement inputs in the formal processes of policy making since the 1990s (e.g. NICE 2008, 2016) the need to 'manufacture' these communities of citizen-publics increasingly became a strategy to "increase the *productivity* of government" (Lezaun and Soneryd 2006, p2) by 'de-risking' future policy choices. As such, the demand to "generate lay views on controversial issues" for policymaking became so pervasive that it increasingly represented "a veritable *extractive* industry" (Lezaun and Soneryd 2006, p2).

This is problematic in many ways. First, these artificially "designed and choreographed" (Lezaun and Soneryd 2006, p3) citizen-publics challenge the very spontaneity of publics formation at the heart of Dewey's (1927, p50) conceptualisation of *publics* as individuals "[brought together by] indirect, extensive, enduring, and serious consequences of conjoint and interacting behaviour". Second, the ever-increasing demands on publics time to engage with policy issues necessitated in part by the institutionalisation of public engagement (consultation) inputs in the formal processes of policymaking or legitimising discourse led to the emergence of divergent and somewhat pragmatic articulations of citizen-publics (Welsh and Wynne 2013). For instance, for professionals conducting the daily business of gathering public views such as communication experts, imaginaries of 'general' publics had to be adapted to the ground realities of operationalising it (see e.g., the challenges faced by the Steering Board in operationalising the 'general public' in the UK-wide *GM Nation?* public debate in 2003 (Lezaun and Soneryd 2006; see also GMPublic

Debate 2003). Operationalising the so-called 'general publics' that are at once a statistically random sample of the population of ordinary people as well as fair, diverse and inclusive – as idealised by Habermas' (1984) model of the 'public sphere' – was and remains challenging. This is primarily because Habermas' (1984) ideals became abstract, unattainable, and mostly unreflective of the combination of ground realities of disinterest and disincentives that dissuade or prevent the 'silent majority' from participating in public engagement initiatives (Lezaun and Soneryd 2006). Publics *disinterest* typically arise from experiences of tokenistic public engagement, perceptions of being 'devalued' or 'not being listened to' or not being recompensed for time allocated to engagement (Ocloo and Matthews 2016, p628). While *disincentives* might range from "gatekeepers blocking access to involvement" and "inadequate information" (Ocloo and Matthews 2016, p628) (see also Horlick-Jones et al 2007; Irwin et al 2013) to reluctance of marginalised and vulnerable groups to engage with authorities or those proximate to them (Canvin et al 2007) based on personal data from such participation being shared among authorities to pursue enforcement action including deportation (Townsend 2017).

To overcome these challenges, Lezaun and Soneryd's (2006, p3) account of operationalising 'publics' chart the emergence (by trial and error) of a process for constructing "interested publics" or stakeholders. This involved screening out voices perceived to "*hijack* [...] true deliberation [...] to proclaim their solidified positions" towards pre-determined specific policy and political outcomes (Lezaun and Soneryd 2006, p9). However, subjectivities involved in such screening processes inevitably raise(d) questions about the implications of entrenched biases and structural inequalities that privilege some 'interested' members of the publics over others such as who gets to decide who is and is not included (and indeed includable) or which values and interests are privileged over others? Petts' (1995) study of the public engagement initiatives that were conducted to develop the waste management strategy for the UK's Hampshire County showed how the 'white middle class' was privileged in the processes of selecting 'appropriate publics' for 'engagement' purposes. Likewise, the UK government's COVID-19 response revealed how the "ingrained conceptions of racialized difference [...] or colour blindness downplaying existing [material] inequalities which disproportionately impact ethnic minority groups [...] inhibited a more nuanced and accurate perception of the [relevant imagined publics]" (Ballo et al 2024, p9) (see also the issues of 'GMNation?' in Taylor-Gooby 2006). In the case of personalised medicine, where treatment efficacy is based on genetic differences and treatment access on whose data gets included in upstream research, (under)representation in citizen engagement initiatives for upstream data gathering has profound implications for equity of access to treatments. Thus, critical scholarship around why some groups have been privileged in personalised medicine research instead of others have been especially critical of

> precision medicine [arguing that it] seems to be proceeding with a monolithic vision of the patients who will benefit from this developing approach to

> medicine. They are patients who are uncommonly tech savvy, highly health literate, self-directed, information seeking, English fluent, health focused, and well insured.
>
> *(Rothstein 2017, p6)*

Thus, the nature of the personalised medicine endeavour has made the realities of operationalising the so-called imaginary of 'general publics' – as a fair, diverse, inclusive, statistically random sample of the population of 'ordinary people' – a challenging endeavour.

Citizens as beneficiaries of public health services and public oversight

In this context, expert attempts to nuance and at times classify and separate publics for 'public engagement' into the 'general' or 'lay' categories as distinct from the 'interested' or 'mobilised' publics (Hess 2015; Lezaun and Soneryd 2006) have been particularly challenging in the case of personalised medicine. In general, the imaginary of 'interested publics' have been widely interpreted as publics that have often had the potential to morph into 'mobilised' (or politically active) groups of interest or concern to the state (Welsh and Wynne 2013). Welsh and Wynne (2013, p540) argue that from "passive non-entities, circa 1950–1990 (continuing)" *publics* as imagined by state actors gradually came to seen "as incipient threats due to presumed deficits in their grasp of science 1990–2000 (continuing); and, since circa 2000, as politicised threats requiring state control". For state actors, 'mobilised publics' not only "threat[ened] technological and industrial progress" (Hess 2015, p2) but also represented untidy, messy, multi-layered networks of multiple *publics* representing increasingly opaque positions and relations that were increasingly difficult to effectively control or govern.

On the one hand, the state response to this multi-layered landscape of politically active publics was to manage both public participation processes (of selecting 'interested publics' as discussed above) and "also materially performed through criminal legislation empowering more police and security service surveillance, infiltration and control of organised citizens' groups" (Welsh and Wynne 2013, p554). On the other hand, "mobilized publics [too have] also contest[ed] the official imaginaries of the public as threat and pose[d] counter-imaginaries of the state, industry, and sociotechnical futures" (Hess 2015, p2). A germane example is the political activism (primarily) against the US Food and Drug Administration and the US state to allow patients to access experimental HIV/AIDS treatments in the 1990s (Epstein 1996). Another and more recent instance is the case of experimental stem cell treatments where publics across the world travelled beyond their home countries to access treatments elsewhere despite, and at times against, fierce recommendations from science communication and state actors to cease and desist from such travel (Datta 2020; Salter et al 2014; see also Chapter 5). Unlike the case of HIV/AIDS activism in the 1990s where people primarily used protest marches, posters, sit-ins, television, and print media to mobilise against the state, stem-cell tourism was entirely different. It drew on digital (social) media to mobilise support and share disease-specific knowledge amongst like-minded patients (and their families) at the global level to help each other make individual decisions about travelling elsewhere to access experimental treatments (Datta 2020). There were no flags, sit-ins, protest marches as in the case of HIV/AIDS activism, just a 'silent' protest by those who defied caution to access experimental treatments. Scholars have argued that the emergence of digital media enabled this new form of transformative activism at a global scale, fundamentally reshaping the 'rights-based approach' to (re)claiming biological citizenship to an emerging form of bio-digital citizenship (Petersen et al 2019).

In turn, self-tracking and various digital tools and platforms of personalised medicine have catalysed new 'activist' forms of knowledge-making and doing in health and medicine such as 'real word data' especially from patient-centred sources. These include patient-reported outcomes, patient-generated health data, medical product/device registries, and condition-specific or disease registries (NIH Pragmatic Trials Collabratory N.D.). Viewed this way, 'real world data' challenges the 'gold standards' of traditional scientific knowledge production by "forgoing the use of randomisation despite its methodological benefits" and being widely considered to "help fill at least some of the evidence gaps" in health and medicine regulatory processes (Saesen et al 2023, p53). This is, potentially, a paradigm shift away from imaginaries of publics as passive downstream contributors to validation and implementation (e.g. in clinical trials, post-marketing surveillance) to emerging imaginaries of publics as (pro)active participants in upstream scientific knowledge production. There is potential for (re)claiming agency enabled by the digitalisation and quantification of the self not only in shaping the development of personalised medicine technologies but also in expanding the diversity of treatments available to publics. However, as discussed in Chapter 3, the infrastructuring of real world data represents a strategic response by authorities to bring such data and its potential back under state, or corporate, control.

Conclusion

In this chapter, we sought to present a wide-ranging picture of the diverse publics of personalised medicine from the perspective of how each is imagined by the three key actors – science, society and state. In the case of the scientific community, public imaginaries differed substantially between biomedical researchers and social scientists. While the former (scientific researchers) referred to publics as 'patients' in literature, the accompanying imaginary rarely went beyond their interpretation *as research subjects* – detached and decontextualised from the patient's lived experience of disease. This was unlike the latter group (social scientists), for whom patient imaginaries centred on the lived experience of disease and patienthood underpinned by reflexive and critical attention to causes and implications of (dis)affectation. In particular, we highlighted the vivid imaginaries of the *disaffected research object* in social scientific scholarship representing the experiences of publics excluded from the benefits of personalised medicine such as biomarker negative subgroups.

This, in turn, contrasted sharply with the publics' own overlapping perspectives of the self. From imagining the self *as a consumer* with agency to 'choose' health goods and services and at times *as a patient* without the agency to 'choose' personal treatment pathways, to the self *as a site of resistance* against advancing datafication, medicalisation and biopolitical surveillance accompanying encroaching narratives of personalisation. While the self-optimising hyper-consumer of self-tracking goods (exemplified by movements such as the 'Quantified Self' or biohacking) highlighted the assertion of agency extolled by Foucauldian imaginaries of biopolitical governance on the one hand. The plight of the patient at the mercy of financialised reimbursement calculi and high prices of emerging personalised medicine, presented on the other hand the competing reality of an emerging imaginary of patient hood, emasculated by desperation and eroded of agency.

For state actors, the struggle was in reconciling these evolving, untidy and overlapping imaginaries of the self with imaginaries of *'good' citizenship.* Predicated on assumptions of communitarianism and altruism, the 'good' citizen was at once imagined as *a contributor* to community 'goods'; altruistically participating in various community engagement and other consultative processes to shape a more socially aligned (and acceptable) technology development and implementation. At the same time, the altruistic imaginary of the 'good citizen' had to be reconciled with the citizen's rights to not only *claim the state's provision of public health services* but also the right to mobilise, politically activate and at times militate against the state when public provisioning fell short. The result, combined with the increasing digitalisation of knowledge making and sharing across government and publics alike, has been the gradual reshaping of the imaginary of the 'good citizen' towards a more informed and politically active citizen alongside a more nuanced, contingent and dynamic ideation of citizenship and citizenry.

Thus, the answer to the question we asked at the outset 'who are the publics?' through the pragmatic lens of 'how are publics imagined?' by science, society and the state produced a reasonably well-defined set of publics, each with its own characteristics and boundaries. What was missing was an immediately apparent common thread weaving these seemingly disparate imaginaries together even though these imaginaries often coalesced in the same person. For instance, the imaginary of the research subject as imagined by science had little in common with the imagined expectations of the good citizen or the imagined affordances of the consumer. Hence, even as questions of 'who are the publics?' produced multiple answers, the underlying 'person' may very well have been the same across all imaginaries. To what extent this is (or will be) problematic for the development of personalised medicine is unknown, although its implications for implementation will be profound. For instance, science-led imaginaries of the research subject will need to be reconciled with and understanding of the challenges of patient access and patient hood as a result of high prices at the point of care. Likewise, state-led imaginaries of altruistic and communitarian citizens will need to account for the vast swathes of biomarker-negative subgroups of their citizenry who are likely to be excluded from future personalised medicine based on their exclusion from scientific imaginaries of the favoured biomarker-positive research subject. Thus, for the vision of personalised medicine to be realised, the first step must necessarily begin with a reconciliation of *the person* in personalised medicine with the *imagined publics* of personalised medicine.

Notes

1 See e.g., "the patient's story [of illness]" in Smith and Hoppe (1991) and in Kaba and Sooriakumaran, (2007). Balint (1964) similarly proposes a thicker doctor-patient relationship whereby the doctor should aim to "understand the complaints offered by the patient, and the symptoms and signs found by the doctor, not only in terms of illnesses, but also as expressions of the patient's unique individuality, his conflicts and problems" (Balint 1964 in Kaba and Sooriakumaran 2007, p61).

2 The UK NHS' Cancer Drugs Fund (CDF) "is a source of funding for cancer drugs in England. On 29 July 2016, a new approach to the appraisal and funding of cancer drugs in England began operating…[providing] access to promising new treatments, via managed access arrangement, while further evidence is collected to address clinical uncertainty, [and] Interim funding for all newly recommended cancer drugs, giving patients access to these treatments many months earlier than before". Available online at https://www.england.nhs.uk/cancer/cdf/?_gl=1*vbseys*_gcl_au*NTY2ODY3ODQ1LjE3Mjk1MTkzNjc.and_ga=2.204063383.600158136.1729519367-854631160.1729519367.

3 "This was a response to part of the Patient Protection and Affordable Care Act (PPACA), which made it possible, under federal law, for employers to vary health insurance premiums by up to 30% based on employee's health factors …[especially as] more than half of all Americans receive health insurance through their employers" (Christophersen et al 2015, p288).

5

PERSONALISATION IN TREATMENT, THERAPY, AND CARE

This chapter will present a range of examples of different technologies and practices that have, in different ways, held out the prospect of 'personalised' treatment for patients. Much of what has been discussed in the prior chapters of this book in relation to personalised medicine concerns various techniques and strategies for classifying, grouping and stratifying individuals based on different forms of measurement, different types of data and a range of calculative tools for predicting current or future health outcomes. However, as discussed in Chapter 1, the label 'personalised medicine' also carries connotations of treatment tailored to the needs of individual patients. That is the focus of this chapter, which considers how personalisation extends to therapeutic interventions in the form of biological therapies; medicines that use genetic modification and/or living human cells and tissues as the basis for therapeutic intervention. The development of these technologies has occurred under a number of labels, including 'tissue engineering', 'bio-based therapies', and 'regenerative medicine', among others, but for clarity we will use the terms 'cell therapy' and 'gene therapy' here. As with other technologies discussed in this book, cell and gene therapies are not necessarily or inherently 'personalised' but they do offer opportunities for tailoring of treatments, particularly in cases where a patient's own cells are used as the basis for the therapy.

As with the examples given in prior chapters, 'personalisation' takes different forms, is implemented in different ways, and has different effects and consequences for different technologies and contexts. While it is only very occasionally the case that we find a medicine, device or procedure developed on a one-off basis for one single patient, there are a variety of technologies that lend themselves to a degree of tailoring or matching between patient and therapy. This 'matching' still depends very much on the techniques of stratification, especially genetic stratification, that underpin other aspects of personalised or precision medicine. In many ways, the

DOI: 10.4324/9781003279556-5

advanced therapies here are the direct successors to, and consequences of, the pharmacogenomic medicines like trastuzumab and imatinib mesylate discussed in Chapter 1. Cell- and gene-based therapies also differ in important ways from conventional pharmaceuticals, not least by virtue of being much more complex and involving living biological material rather than inert chemical compounds (Gardner et al 2015). As such they challenge the established models of pharmaceutical development, manufacturing, distribution and delivery (Umemura 2019) and have given rise to a range of alternative manufacturing and delivery strategies, several of which intersect with different ideas of 'personalisation' or 'customisation' of treatments.

This chapter takes the form of a 'potted history' of cell and gene therapies, beginning with the emergence of tissue engineering and the first approved human gene therapy trials in the 1980s and moving through to the contemporary era of high-cost advanced therapies. It is not possible, within the scope of one chapter, to consider every development, technology, or issue that has attracted public and scholarly attention over this history. Instead, the chapter will use selected examples, from stem cell banking to autologous CAR-T therapies, to illustrate the major dimensions of personalisation, and their consequences, associated with personalised biotherapeutics. This aim is informed by Hannah Landecker's (2007) argument that while studies of specific biotechnologies are useful, it is also important to look at the bigger picture, the better to identify and understand the recurring organisational, social and scientific issues that arise from particular 'genres of technology'. As this chapter will show, some familiar themes arise; the interplay of standardisation and customisation, the underpinning 'platforming' effect of categorisation and stratification work as the basis for further personalisation efforts, and the mutual interdependence and co-production of technologies and their socio-technical environments. As with genomics, big data, artificial intelligence, and other technologies of personalisation, these themes manifest in particular ways in relation to cell and gene therapies, and, as a field that continues to attract scientific, political and commercial investment and aspiration, their history also acts as a guide to the possible futures of personalised biotherapeutics.

In the beginning: the origins of tissue engineering and gene therapy

The technologies to grow and manipulate living human cells and tissues outside the body and to modulate the genetic material inside living cells, all emerged in the latter half of the twentieth century. The relevant techniques and tools derive primarily from the discipline of molecular biology, which is concerned, to paraphrase Hannah Landecker (2007), with exploring 'the plasticity of biological life'. While the various technologies and practices of molecular biology render biology more malleable and subject to greater human control, they are not inherently personalised or personalising. The fields of cell therapy and gene therapy both emerged, separately, before the widespread advent of ideas of personalised medicine. The term 'tissue engineering' (TE) to describe the use of cultured human tissues to repair damage caused by injuries and disease was first coined in 1985, in response to new research coming out of the Massachusetts Institute of Technology (Kemp 2006). In the years that followed, the field gained its first conferences, the concept was recognised by the US National Science Foundation, and the first tissue engineering firms Organogenesis and Advanced Tissue Sciences were founded. These first TE products took small samples of 'primary' human tissues such as skin or cartilage and used specialised techniques to grow and expand the cells into larger tissue constructs that could be implanted to treat injuries such as burns or repair damage in joints. In the main, these were autologous therapies; that is the patient was both the donor of the original cell sample and the recipient of the expanded tissue engineered therapy. These autologous cell therapies are 'personalised' in that, because the human immune system will reject 'foreign' biological material, including that from other humans with a different immune profile, autologous therapies can only be used safely with the patient from whom they were derived. Each batch of the product is 'patient specific' in this way but the expansion and application of the tissue engineered therapy was relatively standardised and all eligible patients would receive effectively 'the same' treatment, albeit made from their own biological material. Autologous TE products are personalised (immune matched) but not biologically targeted at a specific pathological mechanism in a way comparable to, for example, pharmacogenomic medicines.

At around the same time as TE was developing, the first human gene therapy trials were being approved in the United States and Europe (Addison 2017; Martin 1999). Gene therapy uses recombinant DNA, a technique pioneered in the United States in the 1970s, to insert a selected section of DNA into the genome of the cell. This can include inserting synthesised DNA sequences that contain genes not normally found in that cell type or even that species (as with genetically modified crops and animals). For human gene therapy, the aim is usually to add a copy of a functioning human gene to cells where an abnormal variant of the gene is inducing pathology. There are some similarities to pharmacogenomic drugs like trastuzumab or imatinib mesylate, except that instead of targeting a protein or other molecule produced by a disease-associated genetic variant, gene therapy targets the gene itself for replacement. However, for monogenic diseases (i.e. those caused by a defect in a single gene), there can still be many different disease-causing variants. For example, Cystic Fibrosis (CF) is caused by mutations in the CFTR (cystic fibrosis transmembrane conductance regulator) gene and was once considered a prime candidate for gene therapy. There are over a thousand different known disease-causing mutations of CFTR, but a classic gene therapy approach would treat them all the same way; by inserting a version of the healthy CFTR gene into as many cells of the patient's lungs as possible and hoping that the functioning versions of the gene would override and replace the effects of whichever abnormal variant the patient had. Thus, for recombinant DNA based gene therapy, as for so many iterations of personalised medicine, tailoring or targeting goes hand in hand with a degree of standardisation and commensuration.

The clinical application of gene therapy was aided by the isolation of haematopoietic ('blood forming') stem cells. In 1984, researchers at Johns Hopkins University Hospital devised a biochemical method of separating out these 'stem cells' from the mass of cells contained in human bone marrow (Martin et al 2006). It is these stem cells that produce the restorative effect seen in leukaemia patients who receive a bone marrow transplant after undergoing chemotherapy to kill off their own cancerous white blood cells. Extraction of haematopoietic stem cells from bone marrow also provided a step where cells were extracted and grown outside the body, and could therefore potentially, also be subject to genetic modification before being reinfused into a patient. Gene therapy delivered by this method, known as ex vivo gene therapy because the genetic modification step takes solace outside the body, is both targeted (to a specific gene) and personalised, in that it uses autologous cells as a delivery mechanism and therefore each batch is patient specific. By the mid-1990s, the number of experimental gene therapy trials had grown significantly and now included trials in countries such as China and Japan as well as in the United States and Europe. Over 60% of gene therapy trials were by this time being funded by industry sources (Addison 2017, p267).

The bubble bursts: limits to early waves of personalisation and customisation

Both the tissue engineering and gene therapy fields would encounter significant setbacks in the early years of the twenty-first century. Between 1999 and 2004 a small number of patients in gene therapy trials in the United States and Europe suffered fatal adverse effects (Addison 2017). One of the problems was that although gene therapy with recombinant DNA is 'targeted' at replacing a specified gene variant, the mechanism for actually inserting new DNA into a patient's cells was not especially precise and the location of where the new DNA strands would be inserted into a patient's genome was not always tightly controllable. In some cases, the new added genetic material was inserted in such a way as to interrupt other genes in the cell, disrupting their function, and in turn, the normal functioning of the cells. By alleviating one disease the gene therapy also created new forms of genetic damage, which in a few cases produced tumour growth and led to spontaneous cancers.

The popular account of the impact of these events is that these serious adverse events in gene therapy trials shut down investment in gene therapy for much of the rest of the decade. The reality is somewhat more complex; in addition to this small number of nonetheless serious incidents, a host of other technical challenges led to scientists reappraising what constituted a 'good target' for gene therapy (Martin 1999). For example, Cystic Fibrosis, once considered an ideal target for gene therapy since it was a monogenic disease, actually proved extremely challenging. In vivo gene therapy (i.e. where the genetic modification of cells takes place inside the patient's body rather than in an extracted batch of cells or tissues) requires the genetic material to be delivered by a vector, often a modified human virus such as an Adeno-Associated Virus (AAV). These viral vectors have been modified to get inside cells, but to deliver the desired human genetic material, such as a functioning CFTR gene, rather than causing disease by inserting their normal viral genetic material. However the lungs, which at the time were considered the tissue most affected by CF, are both very large in cellular terms, meaning a huge number of viruses are needed to successfully modify enough lung cells to have a noticeable effect on disease symptoms, and are designed specifically to keep viruses and other foreign material out of the human body, both of which factors make gene therapy of the lungs enormously technically challenging in practice, even if the basic idea of replacing a single 'faulty' gene is scientifically and medically attractive.

Just as gene therapy was going through a period of retrenchment and reorientation in the early 2000s, most of the original tissue engineering companies had also filed for bankruptcy (Kemp 2006). Again, there is a widespread narrative that this was due to failures on the part of national medicines regulators to approve tissue engineered therapies in a timely fashion, and again the reality is somewhat more complex. Many of the early tissue engineering firms relied heavily on private investment from Venture Capital firms and they were not able to generate enough revenue quickly enough to produce the return on investment that such private investors seek (Kemp 2006; Mason 2007). Tissue engineering products also relied, in many cases, on hospital departments and physicians in medical specialities that were not used to, or set up for, dealing with human tissue culture, and some early iterations of TE products had to be redesigned after their initial launch to align with medical workflows and practices (Rowley and Martin 2009). Moreover, commercial autologous therapies were often in competition with 'in house' treatments where hospitals had access to public sector banks of allogenic skin cells, ligaments and so on, which were cheaper for physicians to access.

Autologous therapies – including ex vivo gene therapies as well as TE products – also need to be prepared on a case-by-case basis to be ready when a patient needs them. This takes time – culturing the cells to a sufficient volume can take over a week – but equally if the cells are left too long in culture they will lose their function, meaning very precise windows are needed to match the timing of the preparation phase with having the patient ready to undergo treatment. Interviews with clinicians with experience of using TE products conducted by Rowley and Martin (2009) found that the difficulties of timing, and the waste of expensive product that occurred when the timing was misjudged (for example if an operation had to be rescheduled because a patient had complications with their condition), as well as the high cost of TE products were the main reasons clinicians gave for not being enthusiastic about autologous TE products.

At the same time, the regulatory issues for early TE are important. While some TE products such as Apligraf (autologous cultured human skin cells to treat and repair wounds) and Carticel (autologous cartilage cells for repair of cartilage damage such as sports injury) were approved by the US FDA, the process of gaining approval was slow and hindered reimbursement. In Europe the situation was even more difficult and many initial TE products were unable to secure marketing approval from national regulators (Kemp 2006). This is in large part because TE products were significantly different from both traditional small molecule pharmaceuticals and from medical devices (Faulkner 2009b). Many TE products contained not only living cells but also scaffolds of biomaterials intended to give the tissue engineered constructs shape or durability, meaning that from a regulatory perspective TE products often had elements of a medicine and of a medical device in one product (Kent et al 2006). The result was fragmentation, as different EU member states opted to regulate TE products under different regulatory categories with different pathways to market and different evidence requirements: They were considered drugs in Ireland and Italy, transplants in France and Belgium, medical devices in Spain, treated on an ad hoc case-by-case basis by the national regulator in Denmark, and by making a distinctions between autologous treatments (regulated as surgery) and allogeneic treatments, regarded as drugs, in Germany (Kent et al 2006). Such a variety of different regulatory pathways to market, each with different evidence requirements and reimbursement models made it very expensive and time consuming for small firms trying to design clinical studies that would get a TE product approved in multiple European jurisdictions. Yet without widespread approval, revenue streams were too small to sustain the financial viability of firms. These regulatory issues were eventually addressed in Europe through the Advanced Therapy Medicinal Products (ATMP) Regulation which came into force in 2007 and contained a special regulatory category of 'tissue engineered medicines', but by that time the early wave of TE firms had largely gone out of business.

The early histories of cell and gene therapy highlight some of the underlying challenges of different forms of 'personalised' therapeutics. It is tempting to describe cell and gene therapies as at first too novel, too radical a departure for existing medicines to be viable. However, novelty, as Gardner and Webster (2016) argue, is not an inherent property of technologies, it is a judgement about the degree of alignment with existing sets of social and technical arrangements. Almost all biotechnology, not just cell and gene therapies, can be characterised by this tension between being seen as simply an extension of existing medical practices and ideas or as disruptively different from what has gone before. As Martin et al (2020, p220) explain:

> The latter valorises biotechnologies as novel, exciting, and generative of future health and wealth, the better to enrol support and resources. The former naturalizes it as continuing a longstanding sphere of human activity and therefore nothing to excite undue (public or political) concern.

Rather than looking at personalised therapeutics as themselves 'transformative', it is useful to consider the work of transformation that is required to make them viable and where the burden of that work falls. There is a gap, potentially a very large one, between interventions that 'work' in a technical sense, and those that are 'workable'; that is, which can practically and sustainably be delivered in a particular healthcare environment. The personalisation that comes with TE required, in many instances, significant reworking and realignment of existing practices, infrastructures, diagnostic categories, hospital scheduling practices, supply chains, and other elements. The work needed to achieve this reorganisation is typically hidden or minimised in promissory accounts of personalised therapies and neglected in policy documents and media briefings. Moreover, in public healthcare systems the costs of the structural adaptations needed to make personalised therapies practically deliverable is usually borne by the state, and ultimately the public purse, even when the therapies are commercial products.

As the first wave of TE products in Europe illustrates this is also true at a macro level for regulations and regulatory categories governing market access. This is not a simple story of regulation inhibiting innovation. Regulations can and do enable innovation by creating stable, reliable pathways to market and reducing uncertainty about the legal liability of actors producing and selling medicinal products and services (Faulkner 2009c). However, too much fragmentation, too much 'local' (here referring to individual territories within the supranational entity of the EU) adaptation and tailoring of regulations can actually inhibit access to commercial personalised medicines by making market access too expensive to be worthwhile. This is in large part because, although the promises raised by advocates of TE and gene therapy were often expansive, the reality was that personalised medicines typically, and as we will discuss later, perhaps inevitably, target relatively narrow patient populations. This means that commercial personalised therapies need access to large markets to generate sufficient revenue to cover manufacturing and clinical trial costs. One paradoxical result of personalisation in therapies is a push for harmonised regulations between countries: so while tissue engineered products did eventually get a bespoke regulatory pathway to market, in the form of the ATMP Regulation, it was a harmonised, Europe-wide pathway that was intended to be 'the same' across all Member States.

Finally, although it is only one example, the case of Gene therapy for Cystic Fibrosis illustrates how a nuanced approach to dealing with the promise of personalised medicine is required. At present, CF is treated through a combination of new-born screening using biomarkers and genomic sequencing (i.e. stratification of the target population based on prior correlations between gene variants and disease), and can be ameliorated by using a variety of small molecule drugs that target the molecular structure (known as an ion channel) which is affected by abnormal variants of the CFTR gene (Lee et al 2021; Terlizzi and Farrell 2024). There are different drugs for some of the major genetic variants of the CFTR gene, so although gene therapy has so far proven unsuccessful for CF, the identification and sequencing of the gene has led to development of a variety of targeted, i.e. pharmacogenomic, drugs. Was gene therapy for CF a failure of personalised medicine? In some ways yes, because that particular treatment avenue has not come to fruition (although the arrival of gene editing, as discussed below, has renewed interest in a genetic therapy for CF), but in other ways definitely not. The isolation and characterisation of the CFTR gene led ultimately to more sensitive, earlier, stratified molecular diagnosis and personalised (i.e. a selection of comparatively biologically targeted) treatments in place of 'one size fits all' treatment, which has yielded a far from insignificant improvement in quality of life for CF patients. As discussed in Chapter 1, promissory discourses typically emphasise one particular technology, or field of research, as 'the' panacea for many large challenges in healthcare and medicine. This almost always proves to be oversimplified and over ambitious, but in assessing the outcomes of investment of time, energy, money, hope, and labour driven by promise, it is important to acknowledge the unexpected or unplanned benefits than can arise, as well as the failures or unfulfilled expectations.

The era of regenerative medicine

Even as tissue engineering and gene therapy were enjoying their first moment in the sun in the 1990s, new techniques and technologies from molecular and developmental biology laboratories that would ultimately come to replace primary cell-based TE products, were gaining scientific, commercial and popular attention. Following the isolation of haematopoietic stem cells from bone marrow in 1984, other sources and other types of stem cells were also identified and isolated from other body tissues. For example, mesenchymal stem cells also derive from bone marrow, and many organs such as the lung and liver have their own populations of 'adult' stem cells that replenish the cells of those organs lost to damage and decay over time. This is in essence what stem cells do; they are 'immature' or precursor cells which divide to both reproduce themselves and give rise to new specialised body cells such as muscle, skin, or lung cells. Adult stem cells can usually only give rise to a limited range of tissues. However, in 1998, James Thompson and his team at University of Madison, Wisconsin isolated a new type of stem cells from human embryos. Human embryonic stem cells (hESC) can potentially form any cell type in the human body, a property known as 'pluripotency'. This discovery, along with other novel techniques such as (therapeutic) cloning which appeared at the end of the 1990s, ushered in a new wave of promise and expectations for (stem) cell therapeutics. The depleted cell and tissue-based therapies sector reorganised and rebranded itself under the label 'regenerative medicine' with stem cells at the heart of the narratives of revitalisation and renewed commercial and medical hope (see e.g. Mason 2007; Morrison 2012). Human embryonic stem cells, of course, were hugely controversial due to the method of deriving them requiring destruction of a human embryo. However, the intention of this section is not to revisit and analyse the ethics and politics of human embryo research and hESC, but to explore how currents of personalisation intersected with regenerative medicine.

HESC may be the most (in)famous and promissory type of stem cell, but they are neither personalised in the sense of being autologous cells nor biologically targeted like trastuzumab or gene therapy. Instead, other stem cell types lent themselves more immediately to currents of personalisation. The blood in human umbilical cords also contains a type of stem cell, similar to those found in bone marrow. Umbilical cord banking emerged as a new socio-technical practice, based on the idea that the stem cells in cord blood could be cryogenically stored and would be available in future as a source of stem cells both in place of bone marrow replacement therapy for leukaemia and for as yet undeveloped stem cell treatments. There were two competing models of cord blood banking. Private banking enjoined parents to pay to bank the umbilical cord after the birth of a child, so that the blood would provide a source of immune compatible stem cells for that child in future (Dickenson 2013). The other more solidaristic method, aimed to bank cord blood from new-borns in public banks that would make stem cells available to unrelated future cancer patients as needed. Private banking combines the biological personalisation of immune matched cells and tissues with the 'personal' domain of private financial transactions. This is similar to the rise of direct-to-consumer genetic testing and personal tracking apps (Chapter 4) and will also be a recurring theme in this chapter. The irony, as Dickenson (2013) notes, is that umbilical cord stem cells from an unrelated donor may actually be more medically effective as a treatment than using one's own stored cord blood, despite the promise of immune compatibility associated with the latter.

The regulatory approach to commercial (stem) cell therapies, although it arrived at different speeds, was ultimately similar in jurisdictions such as the United States, EU, the United Kingdom, Canada, and Australia. The pathway to market approval is modelled on the framework for small molecule pharmaceuticals. One consequence of this 'regulatory pharmaceuticalisation' (Faulkner 2012) is to entrench an industrial ideal, based on scalable, automated mass manufacturing, and widespread distribution of advanced therapies as medicinal products. Even where cell or gene therapies are biologically targeted or immune matched, the manufacturing and delivery is as standardised as possible so that from a regulatory (and market) point of view the product is essentially 'the same'.

However, (stem) cells are derived from the living body tissues of donors, who are often also patients, and so there has always been some question as to whether cell therapies should be treated as medicinal products or a medical procedure more akin to a surgery or transplant (Webster et al 2011). This is especially true for stem cells that are not 'substantially manipulated' – a regulatory term which sets out the degree of human manipulation warranted to differentiate cell therapies, which are marketable as commercial products, from transplants which are considered medical procedures and not regulated as market products. As a result, a global sector of clinics offering autologous adult stem cell therapies to private patients emerged (Datta 2018). These private clinics typically provide stem cell therapies that have not undergone clinical trials or been subject to review by national medicines regulators, as a procedure, part of a package of personal care that can also include accommodation, travel, and even alternative medicine practices (Petersen et al 2017). As such, this emergent industry has been criticised by a range of actors from bioethicists to cell therapy industry groups for fostering 'unproven therapies' (Berger et al 2016; Bianco et al 2013; Lysaght et al 2017; McLean et al 2015; Turner and Knoepfler 2016) and 'stem cell tourism' (Petersen et al 2017) where patients travel overseas to access private cell therapies not available in their home country (see also Chapter 4).

However, the picture is not so clear cut. The distinctive nature of regenerative medicine aligns poorly with the three phase, placebo controlled randomised control trials which are the 'gold standard' for safety and efficacy of conventional pharmaceuticals (Rosemann 2019). There has been a proliferation of novel regulatory pathways, using different evidential standards, and 'expedited' access routes for advanced therapies including stem cell treatments in both high income and low- and middle-income countries (Rosemann et al 2016; Sleeboom-Faulkner et al 2016) as states seek a competitive advantage in present and future markets for innovative products and services (Salter and Faulkner 2011 and see Chapter 3). This creates a considerable grey area between genuinely exploitative fraudulent treatments and (often state supported) alternative innovation pathways with non-traditional standards of evidence for safety and efficacy, including pathways that support clinician-led experimental treatment (Datta 2018; Salter et al 2017; Sethi 2019; Sleeboom-Faulkner 2016; Takashima et al 2021). Even as industrially produced cell and gene therapies need increasingly harmonised pathways to market between jurisdictions to access a large enough patient population, as seen with TE products in the previous section, bespoke 'local' innovation thrives in a more fragmented, locally tailored regulatory environment. There is also some hybridity, in that different national expedited access ('fast track') pathways for novel commercial products, including those using 'real world evidence' for post-marketing surveillance, can also exhibit some degree of harmonisation since they are primarily designed to support industrially manufactured mass-produced novel medicines. Thus, regulatory adaptation is neither supportive nor inhibitory of personalised medicine per se; rather different models of regulation support different types of personalised medicine development and delivery (Datta 2018).

Both umbilical cord banking and experimental cell therapy provided through private clinics also illustrate how biological personalisation, in the form of immune-matched autologous cells can intersect with the 'personal' domain of private commercial transactions and a logic of consumer choice to configure 'personalised' cell therapy, as an option in a global medical marketplace where access is determined by ability to pay. In both cases there is also an alternative approach emphasising greater solidarity. For cord blood banking this involves unpaid donation to public cord blood banks, a route with little biological personalisation involved, while for other cell therapies, it can involve public sector delivery, for example of allogeneic skin or tendon replacements, or as described below, academic-hospital collaborations to develop 'local' advanced therapies using alternative regulatory pathways.

Stem cell banking for disease modelling and predictive pharmacology

Advanced therapies are not the only way in which stem cells have been enrolled as tools for personalised medicine. The advent of human embryonic stem cells not only reinvigorated the promise of cell therapies after the tissue engineering bubble burst, they also gave rise to new pharmacogenetic and pharmacogenomic projects. The promise of hESC is linked to their pluripotency; the capacity to become any other cell type in the human body. This potential source of human tissues could be used to test new small molecule drug candidates for potential desirable or undesirable effects, instead of, or as an adjunct to the testing on experimental animals that all new drugs must undergo. Here standardisation, not personalisation, is desired, to generate generalisable results. Although hESC do not represent a still-living individual they do have an individual genome, just as an embryo does. Moreover, all living cells and tissues exhibit different characteristics and behaviours, depending on the species, the type of organ or tissue from which they originate, the differing genetic backgrounds and physiology of individual donors, the chemical contents of the medium in which they are grown, the materials on which they are grown, temperature, pH (degree of acidity), mechanical forces, the proximity of other cells, and many other environmental factors. In effect each hESC, like other cell lines, is potentially unique. Moreover, pluripotency, the capacity to become other cell types is less a stable 'state' that can be confirmed and more something that can only be detected after the fact (Eriksson 2016; Pichl 2019). This resulted in a considerable international scientific collaboration to agree and establish standards for pluripotency (Eriksson and Webster 2008, 2015; Hogle 2010; Webster and Eriksson 2008). The issue at stake was to decide which variations between purported hESC were because of genetic differences in the cell line, which were due to different conditions and methods in any given laboratory, and which were actually because the cell line in question was not a hESC but something else (Eriksson and Webster 2008). In this instance, the human biological variability that underpins contemporary attempts at personalisation was a problem to be tamed through extensive scientific and political labour, not an asset.

Despite this effort, hESC have not been widely employed as tools for drug screening (or indeed as therapies). The ethical concerns associated with hESC resulted in a variety of legal measures, from outright prohibitions to limits on state funding and licensing requirements in countries around the world (Isasi et al 2022; Waldby and Salter 2008). However, in 2006 researchers in Japan reported a new form of pluripotent stem cell. Induced pluripotent stem cells (iPSC) are made by chemically 'reprogramming' ordinary cells of the adult body, such as skin or hair cells, back to a pluripotent state (Takahashi and Yamanaka 2006). This technique for making pluripotent stem cells avoids many of the public, and especially religious, concerns associated with hESC, and as a result iPSC quickly took on the projected applications associated with human embryonic stem cells; first the highly public therapeutic promise of using the cells in regenerative medicine, but also their possible use in making 'in vitro' models of human disease and screening small molecule compounds as part of the industrial drug discovery process (Hauskeller and Weber 2011; Wainwright et al 2008). However, because iPSC can be made from primary cells from individual donors they can be used to make cell lines to model cells and tissues with the genome of specific individuals or types of individuals.

This ignited a new enthusiasm for using human IPSC as proxies for individual patients or patient populations. It has been proposed that iPSC could be used as the basis of new personalised pharmacogenetic tests: before being prescribed a medication, a small tissue sample could be taken from a patient, reprogrammed into iPSC, and differentiated to the tissue or tissues of choice such as kidney or liver cells to assess potential toxic effects (i.e. potential adverse drug reactions), or as with earlier PGx tests, to identify 'good responders' (Avior et al 2016; Meseguer-Ripolles et al 2018) to different approved pharmaceutical therapies. Similarly patient specific iPSC lines could also be used to model the progression of disease in vitro to facilitate personalised diagnosis, prognosis or care regimes. As with all tests, the validity of the testing depends on the (perceived) validity of extrapolation from test conditions to 'real world' use (Pinch 1993). Both of these proposed uses rely on the genetic continuity between patient and cell line to justify the extrapolation of in vitro findings to the clinical context. Here, the aim is to harness the inherent biological specificity of different cell lines as a tool for personalised medicine.

At first glance this appears to be an inversion, or a 're-personalisation' of pluripotent stem cell lines after the standardising efforts associated with hESC. However, the utility of iPSC would not be possible without the existing standards for pluripotency established for hESC, nor without the prior work of making biologically classified and stratified patient populations from whom iPSC could be derived (Morrison 2019). Moreover, there is still the issue of how to determine if a result from a patient-specific iPSC line is due to patient-specificity or is the result of the way the cell line was made, stored, cultured, frozen, thawed, or handled. This jeopardises the validity of extrapolation from test to (clinical) reality. As a result, human iPSC have been enrolled in new rounds of standardisation through the creation of large-scale cell banks and registries (see also Chapter 3 on collections of human tissue and data as infrastructure for PM). These banks aim to standardise, as far as possible, the manufacture, storage, naming and labelling of iPSC lines, and set out a consistent minimum standard of characterising data to accompany the lines (Morrison 2017).

Most recently, iPSC (and sometimes hESC) have been used to make multicellular models of human tissues in vitro known as organoids. Organoids again build on the relative stabilisation of iPSC as entities, to build even more advanced proxies for the human body (Hinterberger and Bea 2023). As with their precursors, organoids are not necessarily personalised (for example tissue-specific organoids were used extensively during the Zika and Covid pandemics to model the impact of viruses in human tissue as well as to screen potential antiviral compounds (Hinterberger and Stelmach 2025), but are again being hailed and investigated as tools for personalised diagnosis and pharmacogenomic testing, and are again involved in new rounds of standardisation and exploration. As Eriksson and Webster report

> The ongoing recursive relationship between stabilizing scientific standards and destabilizing experimentation and innovation means that while it is vital to control vitality, this is rarely done once and for all. Standardizing is an ongoing and provisional process resulting from these recursive effects.
>
> *(2015, p86)*

As with other areas of personalised medicine, this has required considerable funding, resources and labour – not all of it recognised – to implement, and demonstrates once again that if personalisation depends on distinguishing between entities, whether patients or cell lines, on biological grounds, they must first be rendered sufficiently similar to make distinctions between entities valid (Beer 2016).

Institutional readiness and miscellaneous care in the era of advanced therapies

Gene therapy never truly 'went away', although the hype cycle associated with the field diminished for a time (Addison 2017). By 2012, gene therapy was making a visible comeback, with the approval, in both the EU and the United States, of Glybera, a gene therapy product for a rare enzyme deficiency. Further cell and gene therapies followed and there is now a small but growing pool of advanced therapies that have been approved in most of the major pharmaceutical markets worldwide (Bellino et al 2023; Eder and Wild 2019). This includes a number of Chimeric Antigen Receptor T-Cell therapies (CAR-T) which are made by extracting and genetically modifying a type of white blood cell called a T-Cell to display a targeted surface receptor that attacks a specific cancer antigen. As a form of ex vivo gene therapy, most CAR-T therapies are both autologous and biologically targeted at specific molecular markers associated with subsets of common blood cancers so they are personalised and targeted therapies. Indeed, almost all contemporary cell and gene therapies are either designed to treat rare disease or narrow subsets of common diseases, defined by genomics and biomarkers. This is partly a consequence of the nature of biological targeting; being 'matched' to one set of biological characteristics such as a gene variant or cell surface molecule means being less well matched to patients with forms of the disease lacking these particular biomarkers (see Chapter 4). However, it is also a consequence of business models that target the higher reimbursement thresholds offered by rare conditions which typically qualify for 'orphan disease' provisions.

Orphan disease regulations in many countries allow longer patent protection and higher fees per patient than for new drugs targeting rare conditions. The aim was to incentivise commercial innovators who otherwise might concentrate exclusively on 'blockbuster' drugs with large patient populations. As Gabe and Martin (2023) argue, the combination of precision medicine stratification of large patient populations into narrower subcategories using genomics, biomarkers and pharmacogenomics, the development of biologically targeted advanced therapies, and existing orphan drug provisions has led to new 'nichebuster' products with high reimbursement rates and tightly defined patient populations, a process they term 'orphanisation'. Many of the advanced therapies now on the market are among the world's most expensive drugs (see Chapter 4). CAR-T therapies such as Yescarta and Kymriah have list prices in the UK of over £280,000 per patient (although the actual costs are likely to be lower as a result of confidential negotiations between manufacturers and the UK National Health Service), while Zolgensma, a gene therapy for Spinal Muscular Atrophy (SMA) had an initial US list price of 2.1 million USD per patient. As these cell and gene therapies come into use, they have given critical scholars greater opportunity to empirically study the impact of these personalised therapies, both at a clinical level and on the political and economic structures and practices that govern how healthcare is paid for (Wadmann and Hague 2020).

Like the first wave of tissue engineering products, contemporary cell and gene therapies pose distinct requirements of existing healthcare, regulatory and reimbursement settings. The concept, and framework of Institutional Readiness (IR) was devised by Andrew Webster and John Gardner (Gardner et al 2018; Webster and Gardner 2019) to study clinical adoption of regenerative medicine. IR rejects both technologically determinist and socially determinist accounts of a technology's success or failure and recognises that successful adoption is more likely to occur when there is an alignment or mutual adaptation between a technology's affordances and a variety of salient characteristics of both the intended users and their organisational environment. The emphasis in IR is on recognising and planning for the inevitable changes that will be needed in any hospital environment to make advanced therapies workable. In this regard IR has been defined as a measure of:

> [w]hether, and if so, how far, an organization needs to adapt to embrace a new technology.
>
> *(Gardner et al 2018, p34 emphasis added)*

In this sense IR points to the restructuring of clinical workflows and patient care pathways, the training and equipment need to be provided (for example hospital pharmacies need freezers capable of reaching −80-C and also staff trained in successfully thawing cryopreserved biological samples), the co-ordination and assessment procedures that need to be in place, the data collection and storage requirements, which are all needed to deliver an advanced therapy in a hospital setting. In short, the infrastructuring of personalised therapies. In a similar vein, Hernández (2025) records the varied range of 'miscellaneous care' work conducted by support staff in clinical trials of new CAR-T therapies, from finding pillows to accommodate a patient with back pain during intravenous infusion of the drug, to staying with nervous patients during apheresis (drawing of blood cells that will be used to make the CAR-T therapy) to reassure them. Both concepts reflect a great deal of usually unacknowledged work that is needed to successfully 'bring the laboratory into the clinic' (Hernández 2025). This points to the continuous' tailoring' or 'tinkering' with organisation and care practices needed to sustain personalised therapies.

These changes can only occur in legal and regulatory environments that enable, or at least allow, adaptation and tinkering. The lens of 'readiness' can thus be extended to encompass national level readiness for advanced therapies, to reflect the need for facilitation at the macro level Umemura and Morrison (2021). Sarah Wadmann and colleagues (2020, 2023) bridge these perspectives by highlighting the 'infrastructuring work' needed to find 'the right' patients for gene therapy, which links 'local' clinical work to regional or national level manoeuvring. The high costs of gene therapies like Zolgensma and Spinraza (both for SMA) and Luxturna, another gene therapy for congenital amaurosis (vision loss), mean that many healthcare payers are reluctant, or even unable, to make the drug available to all patients who might benefit from it. Biomedical stratification of patient populations is often accompanied by, and entangled with, new forms of political and economic stratification as different parties negotiate on precisely who should have access to personalised medicines and under which conditions.

All new medicines are subject to Health Technology Assessment- a calculative process that tries to assess the 'value for money' of a medicine by balancing clinical effectiveness against cost of treatment. As Wadmann and Hauge explain "[c]alculative strategies are not just a 'technical' aspect of regulatory processes [they] are also political in the sense that they contribute to a legitimization of certain conceptions of what a treatment is and how it is valued" (2020, p5). For example, SMA, like Cystic Fibrosis, is linked to variants of a single gene, but a gene that has many different pathogenic variants, some with different manifestations and symptoms. The commercial developers of Spinraza applied for and ultimately received European regulatory approval for a patient population defined by having any of the known variants of the SMA gene. However, in Denmark, the high cost of Spinraza prompted Danish HTA bodies to re-evaluate the evidence for different genetic variants and limit access to only certain specific gene variants (Wadmann and Hauge 2020). When this decision was contested by patients and physicians, the authorities eventually consented to a restratification, including some more, but by no means all, SMA patients in their eligibility criteria. Importantly, economically linked biological stratification can thus be a means to exclude patients from targeted treatments as well as to include them.

In other cases, such as Luxturna, the high costs have been addressed by implementing 'payment by results' regimes (Jørgensen and Kefalas 2017). This means that instead of paying the full cost of the drug upfront, payers only pay a part of the total cost initially, followed by incremental payments based on patient outcomes over time. Turning again to a Danish example, eligibility for the national Luxturna payment by results scheme required patients to meet an expansive list of medical criteria, which in turn necessitated an intense testing and diagnostic regime (Wadmann et al 2024). At the same time, congenital blindness is a progressive condition, and some patients were at risk of suffering irretrievable damage to their eyes before all the eligibility tests could be completed, so in these cases special bespoke payment agreements had to be negotiated between the Danish HTA body and the manufacturer. Both these examples show how issues of reimbursement can not only lead to new patterns of inclusion and exclusion, but also how the decisions about who is eligible for personalised medicines can be (re)distributed among multiple groups; in addition to physicians, national and sometimes regional healthcare bodies, regulators, manufacturers and patient groups can all have a role to play in determining which are the 'right' patients for a particular personalised medicine (Wadmann et al 2023).

Rationing and managed access agreements, while increasingly common, are not the only institutional responses to the high costs of personalised therapies. Some public hospitals, for example in Spain, Canada, and Israel, have used regulatory exemptions to make their own CAR-T therapies for subtly different cancer antigens, often at notably lower costs than the commercially available versions (Bicudo and Brass 2022; Trias et al 2022). Unlike private clinics, cell and/or gene therapies produced locally by public hospitals are usually covered by existing public healthcare provisions and reimbursed by the state. Arguably a more solidaristic version of personalised cell therapies, this is beneficial for patients who can access those specific hospitals, but less useful for patients in other regions or other countries who cannot afford, or whose health systems cannot afford, to pay for travel to receive a 'locally manufactured' advanced therapy. Thus, contemporary cell and gene therapies exist in a variety of configurations of 'personalisation' which span not only different degrees of biological stratification but different sets of social and economic relationships between producers, clinicians, patients, donors, and healthcare payers. Each approach has both benefits and disadvantages and, as is often the case, these are not evenly distributed across society, which is why each instance of 'personalised medicine' needs to be assessed in terms of its particular context and implementation rather than in the abstract.

Conclusion: the future of personalised therapies

The landscape of biomedical innovation is constantly changing. It is important to note that there is nothing 'natural' or inevitable about this; it is the direct result of continued high level of global investment in the life sciences and national research policy environments that incentivise and valorise application and commercialisation of scientific knowledge and know how as a, perhaps 'the', primary goal of funding (Miller et al 2022). The result is not only new biological techniques and technologies, but ongoing and renewed efforts to translate biological know-how into personalised medicines. Emerging technologies that could enable yet further waves of personalisation include gene editing, a successor technology to recombinant DNA (Martin et al 2020), 3D bioprinting (Bicudo et al 2021; Vermeulen et al 2017), automated cell processing robots, and artificial intelligence enabled 'adaptive' manufacturing (Liu et al 2021).

There are a variety of gene editing tools, of which CRISPR/cas9 is the most prominent. They operate in a roughly similar fashion; having a protein or RNA 'targeting' domain that can be designed to find and attach itself to a particular sequence of genetic material in a living cell, and a second enzyme component that can cut out that particular piece of the DNA, replace it, or change its content (for example, changing an 'A' to a 'T' in the genetic code). Gene editing carries promises of greater accuracy (see Chapter 2) than gene therapy and the first gene editing products, for sickle cell disease and thalassemia, have already been approved by some national regulators.

3D printing, also known as additive manufacturing, uses a specialised printer to deposit repeated layers of materials such as metal or plastic in a controlled fashion to generate a complex three-dimensional form. A variant of this technology, known as 3D bioprinting, uses 'bioinks' made from cells and extracellular scaffolding materials to create three dimensional tissue constructs. Most 3D printing techniques use computer-assisted design (CAD) to create a digital template for the object to be printed which then guides the output of the (bio)printer itself (Bicudo et al 2021b).

Robotics and digitally-driven adaptive manufacturing are at once intended to improve the reliability of manufacturing advanced therapeutics, making them less of a manual 'craft' process subject to unwanted variability (Meskus 2018) and more standardised, while also, along with 3D bioprinting, raising new prospects for point of care or 'bedside' manufacturing of cell and gene therapeutics. Each of these developments raises potentially new uncertainties and questions; for example if bioprinted organs are ever technically good enough to mimic human organs, would they then be considered equivalent, and thus not eligible to be owned or patented, as 'products of nature' (Li et al 2020) Bioprinting and automated, digital manufacturing raise new cybersecurity and data protection concerns where patient-matched data is digitised and shared between devices or even between geographic sites (Li et al 2020; Nielsen et al 2021). However, many of the broader lessons from the brief history of personalised medicine sketched out above remain relevant for the various possible futures of personalisation.

Firstly, standardisation is not the antithesis of personalisation in treatment, but as multiple examples have illustrated, part and parcel of it. For most autologous therapies the process of personalisation is more akin to 'mass customisation' (Gilmore and Pine 1997) with a standardised process being applied to a patient-specific starting material, to give a defined product. While each batch is patient-specific, it is not a new or unique product in regulatory terms. Similarly, iPSC are only useful as tools for pharmacogenetics and pharmacogenomics once they have been sufficiently standardised to act as reliable proxies for particular patient populations. Biologically targeted therapies, like pharmacogenomic drugs before them, also rely on the prior work of characterising biological differences and stratifying patient populations into subdomains according to the relevant biomarkers and genetic variants, and of making this information findable through infrastructures of standardised nomenclature and shared data.

With the improved accuracy of genetic therapies, some patients with ultra-rare genetic conditions have turned to crowdfunding to support academic-clinical researchers in developing bespoke genetic therapies that may be unique, or only available to, that specific patient (Regalado 2021). However, even here there is recourse to established standards of accuracy and quality in identifying the correct genetic target sequence and in manufacturing, not to mention algorithms trained on vast amounts of genetic information employed to optimise the design of the genetic construct and delivery mechanism. We should therefore expect the same interplay between standardisation and control, and personalisation and customisation, in future attempts to realise personalised therapies.

Secondly, personalised therapeutics do not simply 'challenge' existing organisational, normative, economic, political and regulatory structures, rather they are co-produced with them. Different organisational, economic and regulatory arrangements enable different forms of personalised medicine. None of these options are without costs, sometimes hidden, in terms of the labour needed to effect institutional change. Moreover, this is not a 'local' issue, or only a macro-level big picture matter, but affects all levels of a healthcare system from national and supranational regulations, markets and policies down to matters of individual patient care. In short, personalisation is never only about the therapy as an artefact, it is always, inescapably socio-technical and political, and this aspect must be taken into account when considering the overall distribution of benefits and harms from any given personalised medicine project or technology.

Lastly, there are more and less solidaristic approaches to personalisation possible. We have seen how currents of biological personalisation readily intersect with notions of consumer choice and access stratified, in different ways, by ability to pay. However, there is nothing inevitable about this. For every private cord blood bank there is a public banking option, for every exclusive private clinic or ultra-high cost gene therapy, there is the possibility for a more accessible public sector-manufactured advanced therapy. The latter reflects the inclusion of advanced therapies in the growing social pharmaceutical innovation (SPIN) movement (Douglas et al 2022; Kleinhout-Vliek et al 2024 and see Chapter 7). These latter points are linked because regulatory and policy decisions can either facilitate or inhibit these more solidaristic forms of personalised therapies. The 'personalisation' in a personalised therapy may be limited to matching or targeting of biological characteristics, but the adaptation of the healthcare environment and the routines and practices of healthcare professionals must always attend to the social, human dimensions of personalisation to make the former achievable.

6

HEALTH DATA GOVERNANCE IN PERSONALISED MEDICINE

As discussed in previous chapters, leveraging increased use of data and health technologies is central to the promised benefits of personalised medicine (PM). As Chapter 1 argues, quantified measurements were central to the development of modern medicine, and (largely quantitative, digital) data remains essential for healthcare providers, not only to facilitate research but also for improving the quality of their services. Technological advancements have rapidly accelerated data generation, conception, use, sharing, and reuse. PM builds upon this growing reliance on diverse forms and data sources, including health data, healthcare organisational data, real-world data, real-world evidence, and synthetic data (which will be discussed below). PM also increasingly entails greater digitisation and platformisation of healthcare. 'Digitisation' refers to information, including medical information, either being manually converted to digital form, as with electronic medical records, or being generated directly as a result of digital actions such as visiting a website, using an app or automated readings generated by medical devices and equipment. More information is available in digital form now than at any prior point in human history, giving rise to the phenomenon sometimes described as 'big data' (Ohno-Machado 2012, and see Chapter 2). *Platformisation* in turn refers to the reliance on digital infrastructures that systematically collect, process and present data through various user interfaces, and is discussed in more detail in Chapter 3. Given this, it is clear that the governance, that is the regulation and oversight, of PM is intimately bound up with the governance of data. Other aspects, including regulation of medicines and health technology assessment, have been discussed in the previous chapter, so this chapter will focus primarily on the governance of health data in the context of PM.

In many legal systems, data is increasingly considered as an economic asset and a pivotal resource to obtain, exploit and further share for economy and society.[1]

DOI: 10.4324/9781003279556-6

In healthcare, such data sharing and (re)use momentum is coupled with public health promises to facilitate medical innovation, augmenting the capacity to generate new findings and replicate results and (ostensibly) enhancing the quality of life of individuals and society at large. This is particularly the case for PM, where a great deal of PM research relies on using data that was originally collected (and digitised) as part of routine medical care and treatment, and which is then shared and aggregated in big data systems where it can be analysed (often algorithmically) to detect the correlations and patterns that constitute 'personalisation'. This repurposing is known as secondary usage of data and is the core function of many of the PM infrastructures described in Chapter 3 (Mourby and Molnar-Gabor 2024).

Nevertheless, the flows of health data needed to aggregate this digital information for secondary use pose issues for several healthcare stakeholders, and entail balancing interests between research, public interest, innovation, patient safety, quality of healthcare and its services. For this reason, this chapter looks at PM from the perspective of the legal frameworks pertaining to privacy (especially privacy of information) and data protection.

Establishing governance systems for data sharing, with the aim of enhancing medical knowledge while safeguarding privacy, can be complex. Tensions often arise, especially in healthcare, where the subject of data protection is significantly delicate. This chapter, therefore, discusses privacy issues in data governance to suggest where tensions may arise for PM practitioners, researchers, patients and PM-adopting healthcare systems at large. To do this the chapter is structured into two parts; the first part sets out the background legal framework, including laws on privacy and data protection, briefly reviews other related areas such as cybersecurity and artificial intelligence (AI), and then sets out some of the main frictions of data protection in relation to healthcare including data reuse, data sharing and synthetic data. The second part of the chapter then presents three case studies of PM endeavours where the practical implementation of data sharing for PM came into conflict with one or more elements of the legal framework described in part one. These case studies pick up on the challenges from part one and again focus on data reuse, data sharing, and synthetic data, respectively.

The overarching argument of the chapter can be summarised as follows. PM is recognised as data intensive medicine. The creation, collection, analysis, storage, and sharing of data about individuals' health are governed by a suite of laws concerning privacy and data protection. Therefore, the governance of PM is in large measure the governance of health data. However, PM also involves sociotechnical change, especially through datafication and infrastructural change. This can pose challenges to extant legal frameworks and one outcome is that PM initiatives can potentially come at the cost of patients' privacy, underlying biomedical ethical values and societal aspects. The cases throughout this chapter provide examples on how these tensions and imbalances of powers can happen, serving as a pointer for increased attention to existing and future data governance regulations for PM.

The regulatory framework for data (re)use in personalised medicine

The first section of this chapter sets out the regulatory framework for health data use and reuse in PM initiatives. This will focus primarily on the applicable laws, which, while not specific to PM, constitute the legal environment in which almost all PM endeavours are situated and with which they must comply. The section will be further subdivided into three parts; the first provides a general description of the major legal aspects of health data governance as relevant to PM, and introduces the main legal areas (privacy, data protection, cybersecurity) which have a bearing on PM. The second subsection focuses in more detail on how data protection and privacy laws apply to *health data*, as this encompasses most (but not all) of the data that is commonly used in PM endeavours. Lastly, the third part of this section describes some of the main recurring points of tension encountered while implementing privacy requirements in health data governance. These include data reuse, data sharing, and data generation. The overall aim of this section is to provide an adequate background for the second part of the chapter, which will then consider three case studies highlighting these main tensions when PM projects encounter data protection and privacy laws in practice.

The governance landscape for personalised medicine

The aim of this section is to introduce the background to data governance as a legal framework, beginning with the establishment of legal recognition of the concept of privacy, and expanding to cover newer laws pertaining to data protection, cybersecurity, AI, and some specific provisions relating to health data. None of these laws are specific to PM, but taken together, they outline the legal environment in which almost all PM endeavours that use digital data in any form will be subject to and thus provide an important reference point for the rest of this chapter. As introduced above (and see also Chapters 1 and 2), PM is grounded on increased datafication and sharing of data between healthcare organisations. Data governance refers to the frameworks, policies, and practices that regulate how health data is collected, used, shared, and reused across policy domains, organisational boundaries, and national borders. As a consequence, data legislation and health data governance become the core elements to look at as they establish the relevant requirements for healthcare stakeholders to process such data.

Governance structures are shaped by different regulatory frameworks, economic systems, and policy orientations across jurisdictions, reflecting the diverse societal expectations surrounding health data use. The processing, use, and re-use of health data have many consequences regarding privacy and data protection. Privacy laws have existed for decades, starting from at least the 1970s[2] and legal provisions protecting privacy, in its different forms originate from specific, longstanding European and US laws (such as the German Hesse Regulation or the US Fair Credit Act). The best known privacy and data protection laws as applicable to healthcare include the General Data Protection Regulation (GDPR) in the European Union (EU), the UK GDPR, and the Health Insurance Portability and Accountability Act (HIPAA) in the United States, the Personal Information Protection Law (PIPL) in China, the General Data Protection Law (GDPL) in Brazil, the Protection of Personal Information Act (POPIA) in South Africa, and the Australian Privacy Act.

Over the years, further legislation concerning data has been added to supplement existing privacy laws, including legislation on open data, public-sector data, data governance, and the free flow of non-personal data. Supranational sources such as the OECD Privacy Guidelines and Fair Information Practices have heavily influenced the evolution of data privacy laws. Some legal systems, like the European Union, have proposed specific data governance legislation to further promote data exchange and reuse: the Data Act, the Data Governance Act, and the future European Health Data Space (EHDS) Regulation set rules to facilitate data re-use from private and public entities, support health data sharing under specific circumstances, and regulate the primary and secondary use of electronic health data.

There are other pieces of legislation relevant to PM that are not primarily dedicated to data *per se* but which nevertheless impact health data governance and privacy. One of these is cybersecurity legislation. Data sharing in PM, when performed with inadequate security measures (e.g. unsafe protocols, outdated equipment, etc.) can entail risks such as data breaches, data loss, or unavailability, exposing patients or healthcare stakeholders to a wide range of potential damages, including the loss of access to data. Legislators have made increased effort to regulate cybersecurity in recent years. The best known cybersecurity laws worldwide include the European Union's Network and Information Security (NIS) Directives, the US Cyber Incident Reporting for Critical Infrastructure (CIRCIA), and the Canadian Critical Cyber Systems Protection Act (CCSP). These cybersecurity laws often establish rules to enhance the security and confidentiality of communications, intending to prevent data breaches or expose vulnerabilities of information systems when data are shared electronically.

As discussed in Chapter 2, data driven healthcare technologies increasingly use AI, so laws pertaining to AI may become applicable to PM as well. These laws may establish data governance rules, including data quality criteria for training and validation of (medical) AI, testing of datasets, bias detection, and correction mechanisms. The EU's AI Act, Canada's proposed Artificial Intelligence and Data Act, and the US Executive Order on the Safe, Secure and Trustworthy Development and Use of Artificial Intelligence represent some examples of current or proposed AI laws. All these laws have been promulgated after the identification of core AI principles, at a national and international level, and they intersect further with sector-specific laws and *ad hoc* guidance provided by relevant bodies.

Sectoral laws further add requirements for PM data governance and privacy. Medical device law, for instance, includes data quality requirements for clinical evidence purposes, so for example a wearable medical device with an embedded AI for self-monitoring (see Chapter 4) would need to comply with both medical device regulation and AI regulation. Clinical trial regulations could require the sponsor/investigator to record, process, store, or handle data so that it can be accurately reported, interpreted, and verified while preserving the confidentiality of the records and requiring appropriate measures to protect information and personal data. Similarly, for advanced therapies (see Chapter 5) EU law mandates that records of the donors of human biological materials be retained for a minimum term of 30 years.

In addition to general privacy laws, the domain of medical ethics has also provided concepts for managing data governance and privacy in the healthcare domain. The Declaration of Helsinki, for example, sets ethical principles to guide medical research. It asserts that physicians involved in medical research must protect the life, health, dignity, integrity, right to self-determination, privacy, and *confidentiality* of personal information of research subjects (WMA 1964). Similarly, the Declaration of Taipei (WMA 2002), adopted by the World Medical Association provides ethical considerations for health databases and biobanks. The WMA aims to balance the rights of individuals to give their tissues or data for research and other purposes, based on confidentiality and privacy rules. Their declaration emphasises the respect for dignity, autonomy, and confidentiality of individuals' exercise of control over the use of their personal data and biological material. Finally, local regulations or codes of ethics may include further privacy requirements and promote the respect of privacy or medical confidentiality. Taken together, we can see that the legal environment for PM is complex, heterogeneous, and often fragmented across sectors, jurisdictions, technologies, and legal instruments. The next section will look in more detail at data protection and privacy laws as applied specifically to health data.

Health data in privacy and data protection laws

Data protection and data privacy laws vary worldwide. Many differences exist across legal systems in how privacy or data protection legislations treat data, including differences in terminology, scope, and broadness of subject matter. Some systems focus on 'data privacy' (as in the United States) while other systems differentiate between privacy and data protection, such as in Europe, where there is a difference between the right to private life and personal data protection (Kokott and Sobotta 2013). Further, the regulated subject matter – i.e. data – may be named differently. In the United States, data privacy usually refers to *Personal Identifiable Information*, while in the European Union, the General Data Protection Regulation (GDPR) refers to 'personal data'. The definitions are nevertheless similar. *Personal Identifiable Information* is "any representation of information that permits the identity of an individual to whom the information applies to be reasonably inferred by either direct or indirect means" (GDPR, Art. 4(1)). Personal data is:

> any information relating to an identified or identifiable natural person ('data subject'). An identifiable natural person is one who can be identified, directly

> or indirectly, in particular by reference to an identifier such as a name, an identification number, location data, an online identifier or to one or more factors specific to the physical, physiological, genetic, mental, economic, cultural or social identity of that natural person.
>
> *(GDPR, Art. 4(1))*

Individual forms of redress also differ. They can be individual or collective and intersect with other branches of law, such as consumer laws (as in Brazil), civil liability law, or others (Zanatta 2023).

Due to their nature, many legal systems consider personal health data as sensitive. This covers much of the scope of PM; electronic health records, 'omics' data and other biomarkers, diagnoses, scans, test results, mental health records, medications prescribed and any adverse reactions, and socioeconomic and lifestyle information as well. A higher level of protection is accorded to this type of data to reduce risks of harm to individuals' fundamental rights. One of the most common risks is the unauthorised access or exposure of health data, which can occur after data breaches. Other breaches of data protection law may entail loss of autonomy and control over patient's personal (medical) information. If an individual is not fully informed or in control of how their data is being shared or reused (e.g. for commercial purposes or research), it erodes their ability to make informed decisions about their healthcare and personal privacy, which as the section on "Tensions in data governance for PM illustrated in three case studies" will demonstrate, is a risk particularly exacerbated by many PM initiatives that involve public private partnerships or the movement of healthcare data from the public to the private sector.

Health data can be 'personal' or may fall outside data protection requirements when considered 'anonymous'. In the European Union, health data fall under the special categories of personal data, specifically called 'data concerning health'. Data concerning health in EU law relates to the physical or mental health of a natural person, revealing information about their past, current or future health status. Health data usually includes information that may be collected in the course of registration or provision of healthcare services, any number or symbol or particular assigned to a person to identify them for health purposes; any information derived from the testing or examination of a body part or bodily substance, including from genetic data and biological samples; and any information on a disease, disability, disease risk, medical history, clinical treatment, physiological characteristics (including height, weight, age, ethnicity, etc.), or biomedical state of the individual. This classification may occur regardless of the source, whether a physician or other health professional, a hospital, or a health device (such as medical device, an in vitro diagnostic test, or other kinds like direct-to-consumer genetic tests). The 'big data' approach to PM means that all of these (and other) types of data can be fed into personalisation algorithms, used to reclassify large disease categories into multiple narrower classifications (stratification) or used to predict responses to particular courses of treatment (pharmacogenomics).

A wide array of personal data thus falls under the 'health data' category. Further examples include data generated by devices and apps, even when produced outside of a professional medical context. Devices that monitor blood oxygenation or heart rate are considered health data when done in hospital settings e.g., to monitor a patient or when a private technology provider provides a smartwatch. It is worth noting that some data protection authorities further specify that health data are also those that *per se* are not health related. Still, they allow for health-related conclusions after processing. Lifestyle apps are an example: measuring parameters such as heart rate combined with other data such as sex or age may be used to determine aspects of individual health and, therefore, can be considered health data (European Data Protection Supervisor 2015). Many of these data are routinely collected for medical care, but in digital form they can also be aggregated and used to inform PM approaches in both care and research. Moreover, the recognition that data collected in a non-medical context, such as via a commercially available wearable self-monitoring device, can still be used for medical purposes reflects the awareness that big data approaches can enrol multiple data types, crossing the boundaries of what is traditionally considered 'health data' to include new sources of information and new technologies.

Privacy requirements for health data governance

Although they vary considerably among countries, some common privacy requirements exist for health data governance. This section introduces the key principles governing privacy. It identifies the most relevant requirements for data governance in PM: anonymisation, consent, the bases for the processing of health data, information duties, and data processing security.

The processing of personal data in some legal systems, including (with variations in their implementation, legislation, data protection or privacy approaches) the EU, the UK, Canada, Brazil, India, South Africa, and Japan, follows certain foundational principles. It is also worth mentioning the OECD privacy principles, which were further implemented nationally by different legal systems. These principles were transposed into national legislation through the GDPR and the UK DPR in the EU and the UK. These principles include lawfulness, fairness, and transparency; purpose limitation; data minimisation; accuracy; integrity and confidentiality; and accountability. As the following section shows, in personalised healthcare, these principles are often not fully understood or correctly complied with. Lawfulness and purpose limitation become crucial for using and re-using health data. Still, in some circumstances, the further processing of health data occurs without correctly considering the purpose of the further processing and its related legal basis to the detriment of public trust. Increased personalisation of health technology often leads organisations to process large amounts of data to create datasets for AI training and validation, which can be in conflict with the principle of data minimisation (see below, the Google DeepMind/NHS case); the same personalisation tools are meant to function with accurate and up-to-date data, which becomes problematic when data are acquired from other healthcare providers, often lacking transparency towards patients (see below Care.data and the National Opt-Out). Integrity and confidentiality entail several technical and organisational measures for the secure processing of personal data, which in some circumstances may be interpreted or taken too lightly (see below, the case of synthetic data).

When health data are not 'personal' data, they do not always fall out of the scope of data protection legislation. Anonymisation is one of the technical processes following which health data (and data in general) are deemed no longer 'personal'. Different anonymisation techniques exist, the main being randomisation and generalisation.[3] However, whether it is truly possible to achieve anonymisation is questionable, especially in healthcare (Ohm 2010). Within the genomics domain, there has been an extensive debate as to whether genomic data, being inherently identifiable, are incapable of being fully anonymised (Wan et al 2022).[4] For health data in general, there is a common misconception that these data are anonymous, while they are more likely pseudonymous and subject to personal data protection.[5] Data that underwent some processes aimed at reducing the linkability of data to individuals – but which still keep individuals identifiable – are considered pseudonymous.

In the European Union, there are different schools of thought as to when data should be considered anonymous. This debate sees two positions: those who opt for a 'relative' criterion and those who opt for an 'objective' criterion (European Court of Justice 2016). Following the objective criterion, data may be considered personal when they can still lead to the identification or identifiability of individuals in any circumstances, regardless of anonymisation techniques used by them or other parties. Conversely, the relative criterion considers data on a case-by-case basis and follows a specific assessment carried out by the controller. Such differentiation is not trivial, as health data, once shared and re-used by other actors, require such an assessment (as exemplified further below in the last case study of the section "Tensions in data governance for PM illustrated in three case studies" on anonymisation and synthetic data).

Processing health data for anonymisation or, in general, for any purpose, usually requires the controller – the entity that determines the 'why and how' of the personal data processing[6] – to consider the most suitable basis. The GDPR, for example, establishes several legal bases on which personal data can be processed. These are usually applied in conjunction with other socio-legal factors specific to health data (Dove 2018). Consent represents a pivotal privacy requirement for health data processing, along with these societal factors and issues that have implications for the legal bases of data processing, such as the reasons for public interest in public health, and the imperatives of occupational and preventive medicine and scientific research (Art. 9 GDPR). Consent, when applicable, is a complex element to comply with, especially when health data processing occurs between legal entities or across different States.[7] Legal consent to (re) use of data in PM research is sometimes confused with 'informed consent' for medical care or research. While they are both connected to patients' rights, they are nevertheless different. Informed consent is a historical landmark of health law enshrined in the 1964 Helsinki Declaration, the Oviedo Convention, and the UNESCO Declaration of Bioethics and Human Rights.[8] It provides individuals the right to decide whether to participate in medical research, join or withdraw from a clinical trial, or use a diagnostic procedure or a specific treatment. In some instances, consent as a legal basis for the further processing of health data is bypassed, such as when needed to improve healthcare and medical research in the public interest. The tracking of Covid cases during the 2020 pandemic is an example of how legal consent requirements were bypassed (Bradford et al 2020). In other cases, consent is not deemed an appropriate legal basis when there are imbalances of powers.

Some legal systems (such as that of the United Kingdom, or the European Union in light of the forthcoming EHDS Regulation) allow patients to express an 'opt-out' for the secondary use of their data, for example, for research. Opting out is a compromise for using confidential data without the burden of seeking explicit consent while respecting the patient's autonomy (Meszaros et al 2020, p99–100) and is attractive in national, large-scale PM endeavours where the value of the project lies in maximising access to population-level data. Consent and opt-out for patients are strictly connected with data subjects' control over personal data. Control is further facilitated by providing relevant information to the data subject in light of the principles of transparency and fairness. Such information duties exist in legislation so that individuals can express their objections to the further processing of health data. However, in practice, this requirement is often not respected or complied with, with sufficient care (as the cases analysed under Section "Tensions in data governance for PM illustrated in three case studies" will show).

Finally, governance of health data, especially its sharing, reuse, and generation, requires consideration of security requirements to mitigate the risks of exposing patients, healthcare staff, and organisations to cyber-attacks. Network and information system insecurity could expose healthcare organisations to cyber-attacks, potentially leading to disruptions in the availability or integrity of data, or even in the provision of their systems if ICT equipment cannot be used (Biasin and Kamenjasevic 2022). Cybersecurity is also an emerging concern in the manufacturing of advanced biopharmaceuticals, which would include the cell and gene therapies discussed in Chapter 5, as these processes become increasingly automated, digitised, and distributed (Guttieres et al 2019; Mantle et al 2019). Security requirements entail executing data protection impact assessments, notifying data breaches, and conducting risk assessments regarding health data processing. Security is also related to pseudonymisation and anonymisation. As the following section shows, data protection issues regarding synthetic data entail a security layer, as they require careful consideration of their nature as personal data, pseudonymisation, and anonymisation.

Tensions in data governance for PM illustrated through the lens of three case studies

Having established the overarching legal framework governing the use of health data, this second part of the chapter now considerers the challenges where this framework encounters real-world PM projects. This section will use three case studies, pertaining to data re-use, data sharing and data synthesis respectively, through the lens of the Care.data initiative in the UK, the collaboration between the Royal Free NHS Hospital Trust and Google Deepmind, and the use of synthetic data to train medical AI and digital twins.

Data re-use

Data re-use (sometimes referred to as 'secondary use' of health data) entails using existing health data – such as electronic health records, health insurance claims, and health registry data – for purposes other than those they were initially collected and is central to PM research. Secondary uses of health data can help identify new disease correlation patterns or help develop treatment plans for personalised therapies,[9] or it can be used in public health and in optimising healthcare service delivery (Carter et al 2015). PM effectively relies on secondary use of data. For data re-use, it is crucial to consider the initial basis of the health data processing and the basis for the re-use of such data. It is also essential that transparency requirements are respected to safeguard patients' autonomy, consent, and control over their health data.

Recent cases have shown how privacy and data control issues may arise for data re-use. One pivotal case is the 'Care.data' programme, which unveiled the difficulties in letting patients decide on the further use of their health data and who has control over them. The story of the Care.data programme began in 2013 when the UK National Healthcare System (NHS) launched the initiative to centralise patient health and social care data. Its objective was 'to improve the quality, efficiency and equity of services' and to allow:

> nationwide linkage of primary and secondary care data in order to identify any unwarranted variations in care across the country (…) with the intention of improving healthcare, by ensuring that timely and accurate data are made available to NHS commissioners, providers and researchers.
>
> *(NHS England 2024, p1)*

Whilst not primarily for PM, the Care.data example is useful because it illustrates the tensions in 'opt-out' measures that also underpin planned data resources such as the European Health Data Space Regulation (EHDS) which have PM as a more explicit aim.

The programme soon became deeply controversial. It was problematic in understanding patient anonymity, did not provide a suitable opt-out system, and according to some commentators, had inadequate transparency and confidentiality measures (Presser et al 2015). In addition, the programme showed a lack of genuine social involvement whether through appropriate sanctions to punish and prevent improper use of publics data, or through the meaningful trickledown of benefits to publics (Aurucci 2023). These gaps undermined the trust between patients and general practitioners. Furthermore, it did not undergo an effective sensibilisation campaign towards the public and, as some authors put it, it lacked a 'social licence' from the public (Carter et al 2015). Opt-out was not available to patients from the outset (Vezyridis and Timmons 2016). Patients were unaware that their data were further processed and shared with third parties for purposes other than direct care (Grace and Taylor 2013). Further developments put in place by the NHS to address such criticalities led to the implementation of a 'two-tiered' opt-out system. In the 'type-1' opt-out system, patients could choose not to share confidential patient information outside the General Practitioner (GP) for purposes other than direct care. The 'type-2' opt-out system was set to prevent confidential patient information from leaving NHS Digital for purposes beyond individual care (NHS England 2018).

After much criticism, the Care.data programme was dismissed and was followed by the National Opt-Out programme, launched in May 2018. With it, the NHS hoped to restore public trust. The National Opt-Out presented some changes from the former programme. Type 2 opt-out turned into National Opt-out, while type 1 opt-out was kept until 2020 and then dismissed. Similarly to Care.data, the National Opt-out provides a service for patients to opt out of having their confidential information used for research and planning. Still, some aspects have been criticised. Meszaros and others pointed out that information available to the public was limited in telling the patients about the type 1 opt-out transition.[10] More recently, the UK Federated Data Platform has led to further controversy over the respect of patients' rights and transparency from the NHS (Good Law Project N.D.).

As these examples show there can be a significant policy push to share health data to foster research and improve the understanding of certain diseases. Similar issues can be encountered in other legal systems – which may show how these issues have a recurring, systemic nature. In Australia, it was the case of MyHealthRecord programme – which aimed to create national electronic medical records for all patients with a centralised database. The programme was similarly criticised on the adequacy of consent, and patient awareness on shared data, security, and transparency over the opt-out process (McCall 2018). Denmark also has had a long experience concerning opt-out, since 1995. Legislative and systemic changes over the years yielded similar concerns, and it was criticised for not allowing citizens to opt out of research participation completely and was described as presenting a "false label all the way through" (Nordfalk and Hoeyer 2020, p403). As noted in Chapter 1, many States have a strong interest in promoting PM, not only as a means to reduce healthcare costs but also to spur national economic growth and competitiveness. However, public trust towards the system could be quickly eroded without careful adherence to consent and opt-out requirements.

Similar requirements are currently being discussed in the context of the European Union, as the forthcoming European Health Data Space Regulation (EHDS) is set to establish data spaces for the primary and secondary uses of electronic health data. The EHDS is another piece of large infrastructure building (see Chapter 3) that supports data aggregation for PM applications as well as for other uses. The proposal put forward by the European Commission initially did not mention opt-out as a possibility for individuals. The subsequent versions were amended to strengthen patients' rights and opt-out mechanisms. The final compromise text, nevertheless, contains weak mechanisms for patients to opt-out as it presents – among other – several exceptions to the right itself and questionably more leeway to private entities in performing public research. Therefore, it remains to be seen how the EU-wide Regulation, once adopted, will be meaningfully implemented across the different Member States and patients' rights respected.

Data sharing

Data sharing is strictly connected with the re-use of health data. Often, the re-use of health data happens after data is shared from one healthcare entity to another. Data sharing in medical research is deemed essential to promote scientific discovery and informed decision-making because few organisations can hope to generate large amounts of data needed for PM analyses (Modi et al 2023). The need to aggregate data from multiple different sources is directly linked to the rise of digital platforms that can integrate different types of data and data from different sources (e.g. from primary and secondary care institutions or from electronic health records and wearable devices). Data sharing can also facilitate AI-based health technologies so that algorithms can process complex datasets, stratify patient populations, predict individual risk, and identify tailored care pathways for specific patients. Within Real-world Evidence and Real-world Data, especially with AI-based techniques, data sharing promises to augment the efficiency of clinical research, discovery and integration, and is one of the ways PM can blur the boundary between research and care, as data generated in the context of routine care is (re)used for research on how to improve and tailor treatment pathways.

Nevertheless, EU data protection law contains multiple requirements which must be considered to ensure that people's information is shared lawfully. Data sharing requires respecting lawfulness grounds, information, and informed consent requirements (as already broadly explored above). Sometimes, these requirements are not fully or adequately respected, resulting in the unlawful processing of personal health data. When unlawful processing happens through data sharing, it can undermine public trust in healthcare services and their systems at large.[11]

This was the case, for example, with the Google DeepMind case, which occurred in the UK between late 2015 and 2017. The main actors involved were the Royal Free NHS Foundation Trust and Google DeepMind. Royal Free was, at that time, one of the largest healthcare providers in the UK. DeepMind was an AI research laboratory founded in 2010 and acquired by Google in 2014. The collaboration of NHS/Google DeepMind began in 2015.[12] Their collaboration aimed to develop a smartphone app called 'Streams' for detecting 'acute kidney injuries' and predicting the risk associated with any given patient (i.e. a 'personalised' risk score). With this project objective, Royal Free NHS agreed to share patients' data with Google DeepMind. The purpose was related to the management and direct care of 'acute kidney injuries', the development of a PM tool for patient safety, and the building of any "real-time clinical analytics, detection, diagnosis and decision support to support treatment and avert clinical deterioration across a range of diagnoses and organ systems".[13] Throughout the project, DeepMind processed approximately 1.6 million partial patient records for the clinical safety testing of the Streams application. Some months after the parties' data sharing agreement, the UK data protection supervisory authority (the Information Commissioner's Office or ICO) found that "there were several shortcomings in the way in which patient records were made available to DeepMind in support of the clinical safety testing of the streaming application by the [NHS] Trust" (ICO n.d.). The Royal Free Foundation failed to comply with data protection legal requirements, which included transparency, informed consent, and a duty of confidentiality. Specifically, the ICO found inadequate information on how the clinical records would be processed for clinical safety testing. The processing was also found to breach the standard law duty of confidentiality as explicit consent for new purposes of data use beyond direct care was not sought.

Beyond consent, another critical problem was data sharing and AI-based technologies, as seen in tensions with existing data protection principles of data minimisation and purpose limitation. As Powles and Hodson (2017) explain, the data provided by Royal Free to DeepMind failed these two principles. The initial data sharing included data about patients being monitored and those who had never been monitored for 'acute kidney injuries', as well as visitors to these patients. It was questionable whether these data were necessary (tension with the principle of data minimisation) and whether it was connected to the declared objectives of direct care (tension with the principle of purpose limitation).

Google DeepMind/Royal Free is an example of how the effects of datafication in PM could undermine patients' trust when health data processing is carried out without informing and seeking the explicit consent of individuals. The use of data was in misalignment with patients' reasonable expectation, leading (as the ICO reported) to a breach of the fairness principle. Such a public-private partnership was not sufficiently transparent towards interested persons (i.e. patients, especially those in control groups, and visitors who did not know their data was being used to train an algorithm that was owned by a private company and therefore could not give adequate consent).

Data sharing between institutions should occur with high levels of transparency and following a thorough data protection risks assessment and impact assessment to understand the relevant legal bases and allowed activities with data. In the case of Google DeepMind/Royal Free, individuals' HIV status was disclosed to Google DeepMind, arguably in respect of the above elements. Such an outcome opens broader questions on who are, ultimately, the persons that benefit in PM, whether the overall population has to make privacy sacrifices to benefit a minority and, if so, whether this can be done in a way that is truly fair (i.e. transparent, with meaningful opt-out mechanisms and transparency). Further, breaches of transparency and fairness principle open broader questions on the role of health innovation and the distribution of benefits when conducting the research entails privacy disbenefits for the wider population.

In the European Union, the EHDS will soon provide new mechanisms for data sharing and the secondary use of electronic health data. Possible consequences of future data sharing on one of the permitted grounds for secondary health data use – one of which involves the training of medical AI – would likely encounter similar concerns discussed here if privacy requirements are overlooked by PM actors.

Data generation (synthetic data)

Data generation and synthetic data have received increasing attention in recent years. As discussed in Chapter 2, one of the risks of big data driven PM is that unrepresentative data sets or data sets that contain sediments of historical bias (for example under diagnosis of minority populations) can lead to the same bias being repeated and even amplified through processes of personalisation. Synthetic data is one possible solution to this, as they can (in theory) enrich incomplete health data, expand limited data pools (for example, for rare diseases) to make analysis more statistically robust, or simulate 'missing' data in data sets that are under under-representative of population samples.

Synthetic data are data artificially generated to mimic real-world data. Rubin (1993) is credited with the first use of the term 'synthetic data' in 1993. In the words of the European Data Protection Supervisor, synthetic data is "to take an original data source (dataset) and create new artificial data with similar statistical properties from it" (European Data Protection Supervisor n.d.) There are three broad categories of synthetic data: fully synthetic, partially synthetic, and hybrid (Gonzales et al 2023). Fully synthetic data consists of a dataset not containing any real-world data. Partially synthetic data is when actual data have some variables changed with synthetic counterparts, and hybrid synthetic data is generated through a combination of original and synthetic data. In healthcare, synthetic data has the potential to enhance privacy. When used with AI-based healthcare technologies, lowering the cost of data access, acquisition, and curation (including cleaning, labelling, and raw data organisation) is deemed helpful (Greser 2023) – again noting there must always be an economic case for PM. Many scholars suggest that it can be used in medicine and healthcare machine learning to remedy the paucity of annotated data in real-world settings or even address population underrepresentation (Kohlberger and Liu 2020).[14]

Synthetic data is associated with mitigating privacy risks; for this, they are thought to facilitate the re-use of health data for research (Surendra and Mohan 2017). Synthetic data could also be used to build 'Digital Twins' or 'Virtual Human Twins'. Digital Twins and Virtual Human Twins are two concepts increasingly used in personalised medicine. They are used to mean a 'digital', 'personalised' representation of a patient powered by real-world data, electronic health data and synthetic data (see Chapter 3). In clinical trials, they are currently studied for future use to create 'virtual cohorts' of patients on which to test the effect of a drug or a medical device (Biasin 2023). Azizi and others suggest they can serve as a proxy for real data and be helpful as more broadly available trial data for researchers (Azizi et al 2021).

Synthetic data may, therefore, entail several innovative research scenarios in PM. However, while they can offer privacy-preserving capabilities, they also have some shortcomings. From a technical perspective, El Emam and others explain that they are not a '100% full privacy solution', as identity disclosure can be possible through synthetic data (El Emam et al 2020). This could occur, for instance, in model overfitting, which happens when an algorithm fits too closely to its training data. If the original data is overfitted, a synthetic record can be mapped to a natural person (El Emam et al 2020, p2). Translated into the legal perspective, the core problem relies upon anonymisation. As seen above, if data is considered anonymous, it is not considered personal data; therefore, data protection legislation does not apply. If synthetic data is pseudonymous or, in some way, there is a possibility to identify or render someone identifiable, then data protection requirements are, in principle, applicable (Article 29 Working Party 2014).

In the EU, the legislature considers synthetic data as Privacy Enhancing Technology notably, the Data Governance Act states that

> [t]here are techniques enabling analyses on databases that contain personal data, such as anonymization, differential privacy, generalisation, suppression and randomisation, the use of synthetic data or similar methods and other state-of-the-art privacy-preserving methods that could contribute to a more privacy-friendly processing of data.
>
> *(European Parliament and of the Council 2022, pL152/L155)*

Despite this reference, EU law does not specify whether synthetic data should be considered personal or non-personal data. Some stakeholders argue that synthetic data is anonymised data (Cristofaro 2023). However, some other data protection scholars remain more cautious and maintain that the nature of synthetic data as personal data should be analysed on a case-by-case basis (Fontanillo López and Elbi 2022). Further developments in European Union case law add further nuances to the debate (Stalla-Bourdillon 2023). Some adopted a 'functional interpretation' of anonymisation towards synthetic data. In contrast, others are more conservative and suggest being more cautious in excluding the identifiability of individuals.

In addition to this debate, data protection practitioners recommend good practices when entities plan to use synthetic data. These include: carrying out privacy assurance assessments to ensure that synthetic data does not qualify as personal data; applying documentation and monitoring procedures, such as having careful documentation of input data and about the process of synthetic data creation; adopting transparency and accountability measures and establishing a clear legal basis, especially when the starting point for generating the synthetic data involves personal data (Murali and Kogut-Czarkowska 2024).

Beyond the European Union's legislatures, other legal systems have also demonstrated further concerns for synthetic data. Whitney and Norman (2024) made the case for the US legal system and argued that using synthetic data may circumvent consent requirements for data usage. Other researchers found that synthetic data may be sensitive to cyber-attacks, and therefore, it could pose a risk to the security of data processing. If this happens, it can also entail risks for AI systems that use these data (so-called 'data poisoning'), causing errors in their results and other performance disruptions (Biasin et al 2023). Beyond the strict scope of data protection, there are further possible shortcomings and risks connected to synthetic data. They could face regulatory uncertainty regarding their acceptability within clinical evidence generation, as there are few standards on how these data could be considered 'credible' when evaluating regulatory authority. There are also critiques of their capability to be a meaningful tool to address underrepresentation and attempts at 'diversity washing' (Whitney and Norman 2024).[15]

Conclusion

This chapter explored the evolving landscape of data governance in medicine and health research. Given the data intensive nature of PM, the way that data use and re-use is governed is a particularly expansive and critical aspect of regulating PM. Two key elements of PM, the platformisation of healthcare infrastructure, and increased datafication, are reshaping the way data is shared, re-used, and leveraged for both clinical and research purposes. In turn, how data is shared and reused across platforms raises critical questions about consent, patients' autonomy, transparency, fairness and public trust, and data commodification raises ethical concerns about ownership and patient control over data. This evolving landscape sees the presence of areas of uncertainty, such as the different approaches to anonymity – see the objective and relative criteria discussed above – that leave open discussions about health data processing. It also raises questions about the role of health innovation and the real beneficiaries thereof. In such contexts, privacy remains a cornerstone of effective data governance.

This chapter also pointed to the main privacy references for health data governance as pivotal across jurisdictions: consent, legal bases for processing, purpose limitation, and anonymisation. On the one hand, these elements are essential for patients' privacy to ensure that individuals' health data is processed lawfully. On the other hand, privacy is a highly individualistic right, of the autonomous and rational self-governing individual. However, the privacy measures discussed in this chapter are less effective, or indeed less able, to consider collective and group harms caused by large-scale data-driven classification, stratification and prediction of populations that we see in PM. Moreover, the strong emphasis on data protection and control of personal data does not offer any remedies for the limits of quantification and datafication themselves (see Chapter 2). These broader issues about what the fair and socially responsible governance of PM might look like will be elaborated in Chapter 7.

Returning to the legal framework for privacy and data protection, the second part of this chapter examined the application in practice of these measures to three 'real world' cases of PM: data re-use, data sharing and data generation. For each case, examples drawn from either past events or current discussions of academic doctrine were provided, which included the Care.data programme, the Google DeepMind/Royal Free and the case of synthetic data. These examples were useful both in underlining the importance of keeping a sound approach to privacy requirements in activities related to PM, but also in illustrating its limitations and gaps. Medical data governance is only part of the bigger picture – albeit a large one. Further considerations, not treated in this chapter, intersect with governance of clinical practice, clinical trials, medicine regulation, intellectual property (e.g. database rights) and further issues. In conclusion, ensuring that health data is used in ways that respect individuals' privacy rights while enabling the transformative potential of PM is one of the most pressing challenges for future governance frameworks. Healthcare stakeholders and policymakers should take note of past cases for current issues and future implementation of health data governance legislation.

Notes

1 As the OECD (2015) puts it, "data are an intangible infrastructure resource that has potential spillover benefits across sectors and policy domains".
2 See, for example, Council of Europe, Resolution (74) 29 of the Committee of Ministers, Council of Europe, on the Protection of the Privacy of Individuals Vis a Vis Electronic Data Banks in the Public Sector (1974).
3 Noise addition, permutation and differential privacy are examples of randomisation. Measures and techniques of generalisation include aggregation and K-anonymity and L-diversity/T-closeness. See Article 29 Working Party (2014).
4 Other commentators suggest more nuanced approaches. See, for example, Finnegan and Hall (2017), who suggest that genome sequences are "strongly identifying", rather than "intrinsically identifying".
5 However, on pseudonymisation and GDPR, see Mourby et al (2018).
6 On the notion of controllership, see the EU's data protection body's orientations (European Data Protection Board 2021).
7 For example, consent rules may vary among Member States in the European Union, and heightened restrictions could apply.
8 As an example, see the DIGIPD project mentioned in Bontridder et al. (2024).
9 For an example, see the ATHENA project in Belgium (Petsophonsakul et al 2022).

10 Another issue was in the use of the terms 'anonymisation', 'pseudonymisation', and 'de-identification', used interchangeably in information material and leaflet (Meszaros et al 2020).
11 For a discussion on public trust and healthcare services (in the UK), see Kerasidou and Kerasidou (2023).
12 According to Powles and Hodson (2017), the collaboration was then disclosed to the public in October 2016.
13 These purposes were declared in a 2015 Information Sharing Agreement (ISA) between NHS and Google Deepmind. The Information Sharing Agreement is available online at https://drive.google.com/file/d/0BwQ4esYYFC04NFVTRW12TTFFRFE/view?pli=1andresourcekey=0-DgTTZSvzRO87cg53HjmPuQ, retrieved via (Tarran 2016).
14 To note, this approach to synthetic data is sometime criticised (Whitney and Norman 2024).
15 To be noted, some laws such as the GDPR may have requirements to address discriminatory aspects stemming from the use of (personal) data. The risk of not addressing underrepresentation and perpetuating bias could, therefore, represent a violation of data protection requirements.

7

THE POSSIBLE FUTURES OF PERSONALISED MEDICINE

The aim of this chapter is to outline what a 'better' personalised medicine (PM) might look like. As the prior chapters of this book have demonstrated, PM is no monolithic entity. It is many different projects, technologies, and infrastructures being envisaged, developed, implemented, tested, and used concurrently in many different locations. Nonetheless, there are sufficient commonalities, especially in terms of the animating ethos and underlying, data-driven strategies, to allow us to make some general reflections and recommendations in this chapter. This is necessarily a normative and a political argument. Our account of what 'better' entails is informed both by the examples described in the previous chapters of this book and by the ideal that PM, like healthcare more broadly, should serve the public good. We reject the popular conception that the public good is best (or even exclusively) served by economic growth through commercial innovation alone. Innovation policy, especially in high-income countries, is often guided by the belief that private control of innovation will ultimately be guided to serve (this version of) the public interest by the 'invisible hand' of market forces. However, healthcare is a universal human need and the right to health is a basic human right that should be determined on the basis of need, not on the basis of ability to pay. Our account of the public good is informed by values of solidarity, shared responsibility, and privileging an ethos of care over the logic of consumer choice. It entails the argument for more democratic governance of innovation and for greater collective input into the design of technologies and the wider systems through which they are produced, made available, used, assessed, maintained, and disposed of.

It is important, even in a critical account, not to discount or underplay the benefits of PM. People's lives are improved, and in some cases saved, by data-driven stratification, tailored therapeutics and diagnostics, and targeted screening programmes. Over the course of the preceding chapters, we have outlined many of

DOI: 10.4324/9781003279556-7

these benefits as well as the potential and actual harms of PM. However, the aim of this chapter is to outline what a 'better' PM looks like, and this necessarily means focusing on the challenges, limitations, and the possible and actual harms caused by PM projects, not only to discuss how to avoid or mitigate these deficiencies but also to present 'doable' measures for achieving better.

Access to medicines, pharmaceutical reform, and a mixed economy of innovation

The economics of PM have been a recurring theme across several chapters of this book. Targeted therapeutics, especially cell and gene therapies for specific biomarker-defined populations, are among the most expensive drugs in the world (Chapter 5). For instance, the precision ophthalmologic therapy Luxturna costs US$850,000 for both eyes, while the precision therapy Kymriah, for paediatric B-cell acute lymphoblastic leukaemia, costs over US$612,000 per treatment infusion. This high cost of medicines tends to attract the most attention, but genetic and biomarker testing services have high running costs too, especially when there is pressure to rapidly return results (Kasztura et al 2019). These financial pressures inevitably lead to unequal access to precision medicine services, both between wealthy countries and poorer ones, and within wealthy countries as different forms of rationing restrict access (Wadmann and Hauge 2020; Wadmann et al 2024). As Sun and Ching (2021) note, access concerns play out differently in different healthcare systems, but they are present in all of them. In Singapore, which has a mixed system of private insurance and state co-payment, access to genetic testing was largely determined by the patients' "inclination toward and ability to get tested" (Sun and Ching 2021, p457) including ability to make the co-payments for access. In the United States, which has a multi-payer, private insurance-based system, the decision on whether or not to offer genetic testing was largely driven by professional guidelines, regardless of predicted clinical utility in individual cases. While in Canada, public funding for targeted therapies was typically available but limited by lack of funding for many companion genetic tests, as these come from two separate parts of the healthcare budget. Thus, "the perceived value of precision medicine is limited by access and affordability, and the type of public healthcare system shapes clinicians' roles in mediating patients' access to precision medicine" (Datta Burton et al 2021; Sun and Ching 2021, p457).

The high costs of precision therapies can also have other effects such as leading to reallocation of finite healthcare budgets, diverting funds away from other aspects of care and leading to 'structural neglect' of equally vital but less glamorous aspects of healthcare (Kenny et al 2021). This can have knock-on effects on PM as well. The Canadian case where funds for targeted medicines were not accompanied by financial support for testing is one example (Sun and Ching 2022). In other cases, even where new screening and testing regimes are rolled out, patients with chronic conditions who have historic diagnoses are often not eligible for newer tests, and so they do not have the accompanying data that would allow their eligibility for precision therapies to be assessed by clinicians (Ardizonne and Morrison 2026). In effect, neglect in other parts of the health system caused by reallocation of funds to PM endeavours can also act to undermine the practical delivery of personalised therapies themselves.

These types of challenges entangle clinical, financial, political, and ethical dimensions and do not make for simple or ready solutions. However, multiple avenues can be pursued to overcome these challenges. Indeed, access to medicines is a global challenge and extends beyond the domain of PM. The medicines we get are to a large extent the product of the current biomedical innovation ecosystem, in which the majority of medicines and medical technologies are produced by the private sector and access to these product is subject to extensive 'private governance' (McMahon 2021) through intellectual property rights, trade secrets, market mechanisms, and increasing capture of regulatory systems by large incumbent commercial actors (Davis and Abraham 2013). In the wake of the global COVID-19 pandemic, in which multiple vaccines to the SARS-CoV-2 virus were developed in record time, but where global access to vaccines was very much faster and more extensive for wealthy countries compared to low- and middle-income countries, there have been multiple calls to reform the global medicine ecosystem to improve access (Geiger and Gross 2024; McMahon 2021; Swaminathan et al 2022; Torrreele et al 2021; Walsh et al 2021). To date, these calls have largely been unheeded, not least because those with the greatest power to act, the governments of high-income countries, have largely benefited from the inequalities of the present system, although there is evidence that this may be changing as rising medicine costs begin to impact wealthy countries as well (Bourgeron and Geiger 2024).

A more 'bottom-up' movement, in the form of 'social pharmaceutical innovation networks' (or SPINs), has emerged in response to issues of access and neglect of rare or unprofitable conditions (Chapter 5). SPINs, as the name suggests, are not a single model or strategy but rather a collective label applied to a range of approaches that utilise, in different ways,

> novel forms of collaborative processes, programs, policies, procedures and/or designs involving diverse sets of actors that break with conventional pharmaceutical innovation practices for the production of safe, effective, and accessible interventions that address unmet societal needs of rare disease patients and that are not primarily market driven.
>
> *(Douglas et al 2022, p4)*

SPINs can include novel digital platforms through which patients may gain access to experimental drugs, novel treatment regimens that use less drug than the manufacturer intended (linked to specific national reimbursement schemes), risk-sharing agreements and managed access schemes between payers and developers, and pharmacist compounding of medicinal preparations for specific patients (Douglas and Grunebaum 2024; Kleinhout-Vliek et al 2024). Social pharmaceutical innovation has also been applied to targeted cell and gene therapies. In several countries, including Spain, Canada, the Netherlands, and Israel, hospitals have developed their own chimeric antigen receptor T-cell (CAR-T) therapies – cell therapies that use a modified cell surface marker to target cancer antigens (Bicudo and Brass 2022; Kleinhout-Vliek et al 2024; Trias et al 2022). They can do this because although several, highly expensive commercially produced CAR-T therapies are available (see Chapters 4 and 5), the treatment uses a patient's own white blood cells as a starting material and novel surface receptors can be added to target cancer antigens and sub-types of cancer not addressed by the available commercial CAR-Ts. This not only allows public hospitals to develop novel targeted treatments for patients who otherwise would not be eligible for marketed precision medicines, but they can do so at lower costs, sometimes substantially so. SPINs offer an alternative model of medicine development, and if supported could enable a move towards a more mixed economy of pharmaceuticals where public and private sectors both have a role to play. However, most SPINs face challenges to their legitimacy, not least because the current innovation and regulatory system for medicine is based on, and thus favours, the model of large commercial developers aiming for mass-market access (Kleinhout-Vliek et al 2024). Moreover, SPINs and other strategies to improve affordability and access to medicines are important, but drugs for orphan populations need to be accompanied by additional measures such as including patient-derived information on whether the therapy improves health-related quality of life and if so in what ways, in both the assessment and prescribing advice of targeted therapies (Lanar et al 2020). Nonetheless the existing successes of even a small number of SPINs provide a basis to argue for increased political support for alternative innovation models, especially in an environment where healthcare budgets even in the global north are getting increasingly stretched.

Ultimately, these issues of cost and accessibility reflect a set of underlying political tensions at the heart of many PM initiatives. On the one hand, governments seek to promote commercial healthcare innovation to foster economic growth, while on the other they also need to constrain healthcare spending as part of managing public expenditure. This intersects with a further tension, between a data-driven calculative, predictive, technology-intensive medicine that requires homogeneity of data subjects in order to achieve economies of scale, and a more holistic vision of care that includes adequate support for public health, 'soft' services like counselling and social care, and is responsive to the situated needs and preferences of patients and public. This more expansive version of care will be considered in the subsequent sections.

Towards care-full futures of personalised medicine

In order to ground the argument for better futures of PM, it is necessary to reconsider the nature of (technoscientific) futures themselves. Most plans for new (health) technology, including those of personalised, precision, or P4 medicine, are informed and structured by the same predictive, quantifying, classifying logics of calculation that underpin nation state's efforts to understand and organise their populations:

> This marriage of forecasting expertise with planning governance creates a decision-making apparatus of a kind that reflects styles of governance that have gradually evolved since the emergence of the 'social state' in the late 19th century. The style of anticipation expressed through these arrangements then diagrams, maps or constructs the future as abstracted and as emptied.
>
> *(Groves 2017, p34)*

What Groves is arguing here is that the tools through which technological projects are commonly planned and organised, cost–benefit analyses, statistical risk-based planning, and so on, treat 'the future' as an abstract 'empty' space into which the needs, goals, and interests of the present can effectively be projected in a kind of temporal colonisation. This recreates the imagined future as an 'extended present'. It is one way in which the interests and assumptions of powerful actors get embedded in projected futures with limited scrutiny, as they inform the design of the very tools through which the future is structured: "Conceptualizing the world and making the world are wrapped up with each other — at least for those with the privilege to turn their dreams into action" (Tsing 2012, p506). Most technoscientific promissory visions take this approach, but PM, with its emphasis on data-driven stratification and prediction, is a future-orientated calculative strategy *par excellence.*

The people in these projected futures are variously configured as the rational self-governing citizens of liberal democracy, the self-interested, outcome maximising 'homo economicus' of economic theory, or the autonomous equal-among-others individual that dominates much of Western moral philosophy. At issue here is that all of these, predominantly modernist, Western conceptions have at heart an atomised, isolated model of the individual as an equal, but interchangeable autonomous unit (Adam and Groves 2011; Groves 2015). This conception of personhood informs not only the modelling of economic activity but also the basis of many of our legal rights and moral responsibilities. The emphasis on equality through equivalence, although arguably well intentioned, renders future people effectively interchangeable, and allows the claim that all such equivalent individuals will naturally benefit *equally* from planned technological futures. However, real humans are not atomised, isolated individual entities; rather, they are always situated and connected – to places, things, and other people. Things and people matter to us because of our affective attachments to them, i.e., because we care about them and what happens to them (Adam and Groves 2011; Sayer 2011). This care is not instrumental 'use value'; people, things, places, and even ideas we know and care about matter to us for more than what they can do for us or give us. If we recognise that we are all situated, connected people bound up in relations of co-dependence, then futures that do not allow for this are always going to be impoverished; another way in which the bureaucrat or statistician's model of the world inevitably fails to capture the realities of lived experience (see also Chapter 2). In previous chapters, we illustrated the harms that can accrue to people who are not represented in datasets, who fall outside the bounds of calculability, whose traits are rendered 'illegible' by systems of classification and the algorithms that operationalise them, or who have the 'wrong' biomarkers to be included in clinical trials of new personalised therapeutics.

In this way, the present reality of much of PM is that most of the goods and services it has produced so far are *not* public goods. This is because the underlying science – centred on identifying individuals with positive biomarkers of an ailment before developing treatments for it – is exclusionary. It not only excludes from treatments all those individuals (and groups) initially excluded from the scoping and research datasets but also misses attention to diseases afflicting excluded communities (see, e.g., our discussion of publics excluded from PM research in Chapter 4). This exclusion, in turn, fails the basic qualifying criteria of non-excludability for 'public goods',[1] which require that certain groups or individuals *cannot* be excluded from using those goods. Instead, goods produced by PM so far are primarily what are known as 'club goods', where access is restricted by subscription, or some manner of (dis)qualifying criteria but without the good itself reducing in quality or quantity for use by others (such as clubs or parks). 'Club goods' can, however, become 'public goods' once non-excludability is established, for example, by improving inclusivity and removing pre-conditions for access.

How this shift in PM – from club goods for some to public goods for many, if not all – might be achieved has increasingly become a subject of concern in the last few years. Many have worried that instead of becoming public goods, the drive towards 'me-ness' underlying the individualisation of health and medicine in PM risks delivering 'private goods' and 'public bads' (Dickenson 2013). Even as far back as 2013, when global interest in, and public and private support for, PM was expanding, the advance of 'me' medicine led Dickenson to lament that:

> I'm concerned that 'Me Medicine' [i.e., personalised medicine] is eclipsing what I call 'We Medicine,' so that we're losing sight of the notion that biotechnology can and should serve the common good. In my view, we would be wrong to prioritize personalized health technologies at the expense of public health measures, which have brought us comparative freedom from the ill health that plagued our ancestors. I see a pattern here—not only a similarity among all the apparently disparate forms of personalized medicine, but also a familiar political formula: 'private good, public bad'.
>
> *(2013, p2)*

Drawing on multiple examples of the advance of 'Me' medicine such as the growing popularity of private blood banking at the expense of altruistic, communal 'we' blood banking in the UK, Dickenson (2013) has even gone so far as to argue for the mutually exclusive nature of 'Me' versus 'We' medicine. Dickenson's contention that "if we take the Me Medicine fork in the healthcare road, we can't simultaneously go down the We Medicine route" is, however, perhaps unnecessarily bleak and has been challenged by subsequent accounts discussed next.

Solidarity and patient-centred care

Prainsack's suggestion of "a solidarity-based approach [with] a focus on health care that is affordable and accessible for all" argues against a zero-sum conceptualisation of 'We-vs-Me' to argue for "a kind of personalized medicine that does not force us to choose between 'Me Medicine' and 'We Medicine'" (2017b, p35). Rather, Prainsack conceptualises solidarity "as a practice expressing the commitment to accept costs to help others with whom we recognize similarity in a relevant respect" (2017b, p35). Here Prainsack draws on the notion of relational autonomy found both in legal and feminist scholarship. Legal scholars argue that "[w]hat actually makes human autonomy possible is not isolation but relationship" (Nedelsky 1990, p169), while feminist scholars emphasise "receptiveness to connectedness, to the recognition that human life is impossible without nurturing from those who care for us when we are helpless and dependent" (Radin 1996, p72). Extrapolated to the wider healthcare apparatus, this conceptualisation raises the question that:

> [I]f persons are seen as relational beings whose boundaries are porous, can we isolate the benefit and well-being of some from the fate of others? If we conclude—as I suggest—that we cannot, would this not lead us to supporting universal health care that is accessible and affordable for all?
>
> *(Prainsack 2017b, p35)*

The answer is a transformative rethinking of the organising logic based on the atomised, self-interested rational individual, in favour of a 'relational' one. Solidarity is intended as a counterpoint and corrective to the self-interested' individualism of neoliberal consumerist approaches to healthcare and as such has an arguably European heritage (e.g. Sun and Ching [2021] note that European-style universal healthcare coverage is effectively impossible in the United States). There are several ways in which such a relational and situated model of persons can inform and guide a model of 'better' PM. One is patient-centred care. In its fullest formulation patient-centred care:

> (a) explores the patients' main reason for the visit, concerns, and need for information; (b) seeks an integrated understanding of the patients' world—that is, their whole person, emotional needs, and life issues; (c) finds common ground on what the problem is and mutually agrees on management; (d) enhances prevention and health promotion; and (e) enhances the continuing relationship between the patient and the doctor.
>
> *(Stewart 2001, p445)*

The link to our discussion so far is the emphasis on considering the patient as a "whole person [with] emotional needs, and life issues" rather than focusing solely or mainly on data points, biomarkers, and diagnostic or risk-based classifications. This explicitly acknowledges the situatedness of patients in a lifeworld and a social context and ideally recognises them as people whose relationships to other people, places, ideas, and things matters and can be taken into account when making medical decisions. Care is always necessarily more than choice. In Chapter 4, we discussed how choice, and the growing imperative to take responsibility for one's own health and wellbeing (again as an atomised individual) – and indeed for the wellbeing of (future) children – can be a burden.

Too much of an emphasis or reliance on informed choice as a way of managing decisions about tests and treatments can also lead to problems with over-diagnosis and a transfer of responsibility from physicians to patients in a way that causes anxiety and feelings of guilt or regret for patients experiencing the 'diagnostic cascade' that follows. It is also well documented that an individual's capacity to choose is limited by a range of cognitive, health, and psychosocial factors, so choice does not provide a 'level playing field' in the battle for health (Kerr et al 2018).

Here, choice, although configured as a tool of personal empowerment, is shown to exhibit a lack of care. Choice alone fails to attend to the vulnerabilities, needs, and values of the situated, whole person who may or may not have the time, the resources, the social support network, or the capabilities to 'make informed healthy lifestyle choices' and who may or may not have the emotional resilience or be in an appropriate cultural and moral context to assume ethical responsibilities in the face of the healthcare profession's abrogation of decisions about who lives and who dies (Kelly 2009). In patient-centred care, by contrast, the emphasis on discussing the patient's concerns and reaching a mutually agreed way forward is intended to alleviate at least some of the burden of anxiety and uncertainty that can come from being faced with a range of options and choices, without returning to an era of physicians paternalistically imposing a solution on the patient. Patient-centred care is distinct from PM, although one of the critiques of the term 'personalised medicine' is that it can misleadingly suggest to patients that what is being offered by PM will involve a more holistic conception of the patient as person (Budin-Ljøsne and Harris 2016). However, this does not mean that patient-centred care is inimical to PM.

Patient-centred care is often extended beyond patient–practitioner interactions by, and delivered through, Patient and Public Involvement and Engagement. 'Involvement' here refers to incorporation of users of healthcare services into the planning, delivery, and evaluation of those services (Forbat 2009). The 'engagement' in Patient and Public Involvement and Engagement is conceptualised as "a further development, referring to working in partnership with service-users having them inform (i) service redesign/improvement, (ii) policy, (iii) research and (iv) their own care/treatment" (Forbat 2009, p84). Using the example of artificial intelligence tools in predicting mental health outcomes, Skorburg et al (2024) argue that an ethos of patient participation and involvement clearly *can* be in tension with data-driven PM technologies. However, this partly results from the developers and designers of digital PM tools being removed from, and unfamiliar with, the lived experiences of mental health patients and service users. As such, the design of such tools largely fails to leave room for the patient voice and embeds "tendencies toward treating participants as data points that arise when AI/ML methods are utilized in mental health research" (Skorburg et al 2024, p145). Those same authors also recommend that greater involvement of mental health service users in the design of digital tools, and greater scope for allowing patient feedback on how such tools are used in practice (including how the data is stored, accessed, transferred, etc.) could reduce the depersonalisation all too common in the data-driven calculations of PM.

As with public engagement, discussed in Chapter 4, these endeavours can, if undertaken cynically, be little more than window dressing, but if patients are able to be directly involved in making meaningful decisions about the organisation and delivery of their care, then real benefits can be achieved. For example, the RUDY (Rare UK Diseases of bone, joints, and blood vessels) study was designed with patient participation built into its organisational model (Teare et al 2017). RUDY uses online questionnaires and other digital tools to capture longitudinal data on patients' quality of life, the frequency of bone fractures, and related data. The patient-centredness emerges through the direct collaboration of the research and clinical teams with a patient forum in designing the platform and its components:

> A balance is struck between which data the researchers are interested in, and what makes sense for the participants. For example, enabling participants to provide a label for fracture events, such as 'sister's birthday' to ensure that they can also use the platform for their own benefit, rather than just setting up a research database to record the 'fractured tibia'.
>
> *(Teare et al 2017, p819)*

This is one small example of patient-centred involvement, and not specific to PM. However, the relevance of the RUDY study as an exemplar of what can be done is bolstered because it occurs in the context of rare disease where, just as in much of PM, the boundaries between care and research are increasingly blurred. Beyond this example, a more participatory PM necessarily allows for a broader calculus of 'what matters'.

Responsible research and innovation: better publics of PM?

In the first chapter of this book, we introduced the idea that PM, in all its guises and iterations, is animated by promise. The aspiration that drives different groups of people in different countries around the world to work on projects of PM is at base, the hope of better future healthcare. However, in the same chapter, we also made it clear that imagined or projected futures are also political. At stake is whose idea of 'better' is being advanced and implemented, who (and what) is, and is not, included in these projected futures, which interests are served and which are marginalised or silenced, and who gets to decide? The power to articulate and advance sociotechnical futures is not equally distributed (Groves 2016; Tsing 2012). Some voices and interests are much more prominent and powerful than others. Promissory visions typically start out broad and vaguely defined. The details of exactly how implementation of what was promised will be achieved, and what the resulting sociotechnical arrangement will look like, are commonly worked out iteratively and somewhat experimentally through the process of development and delivery. This creates indeterminacy, which is why what is delivered may not match with what was expected by all parties. This is especially the case when different values and aims come into conflict in the course of developing and implementing the large-scale infrastructures needed to deliver PM, as discussed in Chapter 3.

When considering technological projects such as PM programmes we must always ask *qui bono* – who benefits? Are benefits to some groups, for example in the form of market growth and profit, achieved at the expense of promised benefits to other groups (perhaps patients or taxpayers)? Several chapters have discussed the idea that PM requires a restructuring and reorganisation of medicine, and of health services more broadly, whether this was framed through the lens of building Institutional Readiness for novel therapeutics (Chapter 5), the labour of developing and maintaining new digital and physical infrastructures of PM (Chapter 3) or simply the ongoing professional work of caring for patients in a changing healthcare environment. In countries with a public healthcare system, much of this work is undertaken by the public sector, which also bears much of the economic cost of reorganisation, upskilling and infrastructuring. However, since PM is always also a business model (Chapter 2), the financial rewards of adopting new technologies may, especially in the short to medium term, accrue more to the private sector companies that develop and own these PM technologies than to patients, the public or public sector healthcare organisations and their staff. This is especially the case where technology platforms, such as digital services, can be configured as proprietary rent-generating assets that extract revenue (and often data) from public sector health services on an ongoing basis (Birch 2017).

Initiatives to promote more responsible innovation often focus on 'upstream' (i.e. at the early stages of technology development) engagement with relevant stakeholder groups (Kerr et al 2018 and see Chapter 4). However, any scientist's agency and capacity to make ethically informed decisions are limited both by the scope of their knowledge and by the distribution of responsibility among multiple parties. Any technological artefact is necessarily "part of a long chain of people, products, tools, machines, money, and so forth" (Akrich 1992, p205). Modern industrial technologies in particular are typically subject to multiple, complex, and overlapping inputs and assessments during the design and implementation phases. Focusing on any one type of actor minimises;

> the extent to which persistent inequities or injustices are not unfortunate consequences of an individual action that could or should be corrected, but rather *systemic features of the environment in which technologies are developed*, including the environment specific to small start-up companies, which is heavily influenced by the competitive dynamics of the business environment.
>
> *(Powell et al 2022, p4–5, emphasis added)*

As discussed in Chapter 4, engagement related to Responsible Research and Innovation exercises tends to favour selected 'publics' that are wealthier and more articulate, and, at worst, can be co-opted to produce 'stage-managed' shows of superficial 'public support' for new technologies. These often focus narrowly on established risks and benefits of the technology without allowing consideration of wider social and environmental impacts. As Kerr et al argue, redressing this:

> requires that we consider the role of the market in addressing and generating vulnerabilities and what this means for responsible innovation. We also need to consider how the market provides technological solutions to want and disease via innovations sold as commodities and how these processes can generate vulnerabilities because they distribute resources unevenly on the basis of ability to consume not on the basis of need.
>
> *(2018, p26)*

These insights direct us to understand that efforts to foster a better, more democratically governed, socially responsible PM, need to take account of the business of medical innovation. Technological innovations, including novel technologies of PM, are produced by complex, distributed ecosystems of actors including academics, small businesses, large incumbent multinational corporations, regulatory agencies, research ethics oversight bodies, health technology assessment agencies, venture capital firms and other investors, healthcare markets, hospital managers, physicians and other healthcare professions, university technology transfer offices, patent attorneys, insurance companies, and others. In keeping with the model of meaningful patient and public involvement and engagement (PPIE) as a corrective for some of the local harms of PM in clinical encounters, responsible consultation, and dialogue with the publics of PM must allow debate about a similarly broad range of topics from the environmental impacts of data-driven medicine (Samuel and Lucassen 2022) to the impact on health service budgets of 'hidden' restructuring costs embedded in PM or the diversion of funds from existing services to pay for new PM services, and the custodianship of medical and health data. As with the example of AI in mental health services, addressing the situated needs of individuals and communities requires ongoing attention, not just a one-off consultation. Continuous dialogue and engagement with all users and patients, not just the vocal, well-resourced, or privileged ones, allows for new issues to become known and for input from participation to feedback into the oversight of PM, including challenging the nature and extent of the 'private governance' to which PM is subject (McMahon 2021), as well as the shaping the design and use of PM systems. This requires PM infrastructures that are *capable* of supporting participation and being adapted, even restructured, in response to feedback.

Solidarity and data governance

An ethos of solidarity can also be extended to considerations of how the personal data that drives so much of PM can be governed. One option is dynamic consent. Dynamic consent is a suite of digital tools that allow patients or research participants to apply a more granular level of control over how their personal data are used and which parties can have access, and to change this over time (Kaye et al 2015). Dynamic consent can also facilitate updating participants about research outcomes, return of test results, and management of incidental findings (Lay et al 2024). At first glance, dynamic consent appears to favour choice over care, and indeed one of the frequent criticisms levelled at dynamic consent is that patients and participants will be overwhelmed by a plethora of trivial choices, resulting in 'consent fatigue' (Steinsbekk et al 2013). However, this stance stems from a failure to properly understand the full scope of dynamic consent. The granular consent preferences were only ever meant to be one tool in a broader digital platform that would ultimately enable greater dialogue between patients and healthcare professionals or scientists with the aim of making consent more informed and more genuinely participatory (Teare et al 2015, 2021). Beyond consent, Prainsack (2017b) suggests that the logic of relational autonomy should serve as the basis for shaping health data governance, replacing the current focus on "atomistic individual autonomy [which] has led to efforts being channelled into increasing individual control over health data use at the cost of expanding collective ownership and oversight" (p35).

Incremental progress towards solidaristic approaches can be seen across a range of recent efforts in PM. One such effort centres on improving cross-national access to and interoperability of a diverse pool of genetic data currently stored across nationally and locally held data repositories, biobanks, registries, and so on, but where access is protected under the data protection rules of each jurisdiction (see, e.g., our discussion of the implications of data protection in Chapter 6). For instance, a cross-national collaboration agreement between Canada and Europe for "human data storage, integration and sharing to enable personalised medicine approaches" aims "to enhance and standardise data deposition, curation and exchange procedures thus ensuring better data reuse and increased benefit to the scientific communities worldwide" (European Commission 2017). Numerous projects funded under this collaborative agreement are aimed at expanding access to diverse cross-national patient data for PM research. Examples of projects include the EUCAN-Connect (2019) project, described as "a federated FAIR platform enabling large-scale analysis of high-value cohort data connecting Europe and Canada in personalized health", and the CINECA project (N.D.), which aims to establish a "Common Infrastructure for National Cohorts in Europe, Canada, and Africa". The primary aim here is to make PM research more inclusive and accessible by providing access to geographically and demographically diverse research datasets, although as noted in Chapter 2, improving diversity in data sets is not simply a matter of more data but the *right* data for the questions being asked (Global Alliance for Genomics and Health 2024).

While these initiatives are undeniably steps in the right direction, so far they represent little more than data-sharing coalitions between advanced economies. To what extent these data-sharing coalitions will coalesce into meaningful solidarities, tied together by pragmatic and doable actions needed to deliver 'we' medicine beyond underspecified abstract ideals, remains to be seen. 'Doable actions' suggest concrete steps such as

> strengthening harm mitigation instruments to ensure that people who are harmed by data use have effective remedies—which the legal system does not always provide—as well as placing more emphasis on whether or not data use is in the public interest.
>
> *(Prainsack 2017b, p35)*

'Public interest', understood here as the delivery of public (instead of club) goods in PM, is envisioned as encapsulating calls for regulatory simplification to enable 'easier' access to and (re)use of data goods for public benefit as well as setting up the 'collective control and oversight' of the data goods thus produced (Prainsack and Kickbusch 2024). In turn, doable actions are intended to take forward and protect the 'public interest' through collective control and oversight aimed at mitigating harms (Prainsack 2017b). These include a range of measures. Key among these are legal and enforceable measures to identify risks of harms (e.g., through risk assessments) not only to the individual but also, and perhaps more importantly, assessing risks to the collective including secondary data subjects (Prainsack 2017b) who might not themselves be data owners but might nevertheless be indirectly impacted by data (re)use (Prainsack and Kickbusch 2024). For instance, PM developed using the readily available data of populations in Western Europe, when deployed in non-European locations might not benefit local public health needs but will still require the expenditure of scarce public health resources that could have been better used elsewhere, thus negatively impacting local populations (i.e., the secondary data subjects). Thus, measures assessing and integrating the risk of harms to the wider collective (or 'we' medicine), beyond harms to the individual (or 'me' medicine), is key to the public interest.

Privacy and data protection are configured in European and US law as primarily individual rights (Kammourieh et al 2016; Mantelero 2016). Although data protection laws, such as the EU GDPR, place specific safeguards on processing data pertaining categories such as gender, ethnicity, and political, religious, or sexual orientations, the use of these categories can still creep into PM, either through the presence of unrecognised proxy measures in datasets or because of inferred links between, for example, the incidence of particular biological markers and specific populations, as with racial categories and genetic data. This can lead to group harms where an individual does not have to be directly identified in order to be allocated to a category associated with stigmatisation or discrimination. Not all such actions are harmful, of course; equity-based public health, for example, requires positively discriminating between groups to allocate greater resources to those with greatest need (Asgarinia 2024). However, the potential for harm has led some legal scholars to advocate for an additional layer of group privacy to prevent collective harms through data-driven discrimination (Floridi 2014; Kammourieh et al 2016; Mantelero 2016). To date, privacy-based arguments for recognising group harms have had limited legal impact, although where groups are recognised, by their members and by external parties as a community, there is scope for modes of group protection other than those grounded in privacy law. For example, many communities, particularly First Nations and Aboriginal communities, as well as heavily researched neighbourhoods and LGBTQI communities, have put measures in place to govern how data about them is collected and used (Doerksen et al 2024). These range from guidelines on community engagement to community advisory and research review boards who negotiate terms of access to community members as research participants and data subjects. Patient groups and charities also increasingly play a role in both advocating for specific health research, negotiating terms of data collection and (re)use, and even creating their own data repositories (Callon and Rabeharisoa 2008; Terry et al 2007). These models of collective action offer one route to redress the power imbalance between patients or members of the public who are data subjects and the large corporations or nation states who have access to the accumulated data sets.

In an era of 'big data', pattern recognition algorithms can create new classifications not based on traditional measures or labels, which even the data scientists who use such programmes may not be aware of, but which can nonetheless provide the basis for taking actions that affect these new collectives (Mantelero 2016). The same risks of group harms apply, but here both privacy laws and collective action strategies are of limited use as members of data-defined collectives are themselves unlikely to be aware of the grouping or consider themselves members of a group (Asgarinia 2024). Nonetheless, even here some recommendations of group privacy advocates have merit in creating fairer PM, including giving national data protection authorities greater power to consider group harms in their assessments, mandating more stringent privacy-by-design measures on organisations developing data-driven PM services, and fostering stronger international norms that acknowledge group harms as a form of unwarranted discrimination. Yet another doable action is to put in place (re)distributive measures such as taxation or other similar fiscal tools to enable and oversee a fair and democratised distribution of the considerable 'commercial gains' from public data use that have so far overwhelmingly accrued to commercial actors (Prainsack and Kickbusch 2024). Following from this, El-Sayed et al (2023) conceptualise a shift away from assessing data goods based on public *interest* to assessing their public *value* that consider multiple factors from oversight arrangements to risk assessments that consider secondary data subjects.

Conclusions: a human personalised medicine is a question of scale

It is a truism in Science and Technology Studies that things could always be otherwise, albeit only with sufficient work. Many versions of PM are possible, and these can deliver greater or lesser public good. The aims of this final chapter have been to identify ways to steer current and future PM projects towards the former. We agree with Prainsack (2017b) that a PM approach, which balances a focus on stratification and distinction with a focus on collective wellbeing and the common good, is both possible and desirable. The capacity to use data that depend on fine-grained differentiation between people, and between groups, is most beneficial when informed by equity, that is, when conducted with the aim of giving the greatest attention to those with the greatest need. However, logics of quantification, measurement, and calculation are inherently abstracting from social context. The scale, or more accurately the scalability, of PM, as evidenced in the vast national and international infrastructure building projects (Chapter 3) necessarily requires homogenisation of data types. In order to be compared, measured, ranked, and distinguished, people and populations must first be rendered sufficiently similar to be comparable (Beer 2016; Tsing 2012). The greater the scale of specific PM endeavours, the greater the potential for context insensitivity and the resulting harms of exclusion, illegibility, and discrimination that we have set out in this chapter and throughout this book.

The solutions that we propose also engage with this question of scalability. SPINs, for example, are local or regional networks that take a bottom-up approach to trying to make certain medicines available more affordably and/or for neglected populations in particular contexts. Solidaristic approaches to data governance (popularly referred as data solidarity) recognise collective goods and the potential for collective as well as merely individual harms, and various forms of shared oversight of data access or data use can be expended on and supplemented. Moreover, we suggest that solidaristic approaches can be extended to other upstream and downstream phases of the PM discovery and development pipeline. For instance, a global map "illustrating the diversity of 60 precision medicine initiatives across the globe" revealed an expected concentration of initiatives in North America and

Europe with only a handful in the rest of the word (Baird et al 2023, p4). To meaningfully democratise access at the global level, what is needed are measures aimed at developing PM that target local unmet needs. This can be achieved through solidaristic approaches focused on building global capacity for PM research by supporting the expansion of national and local centres for PM research. Such local or regional centres can help locally-based researchers more readily access genetic data (biomarkers) representative of relevant populations typically protected national or community laws and regulations, by working within these data protection frameworks to develop local solutions for local disease needs. Here, doable actions that foster North–South and South–South collaborations around knowledge exchange, as well as infrastructural and capacity-building grants, would go a long way towards meaningfully democratising access. Part of any change towards a more equitable orientation of global research priorities must require new infrastructures that allow and support such work. One attempt at building this kind of infrastructure is the ISIDORe consortium (N.D.). It is intended to facilitate research priority setting by under resourced actors by mobilising a collaboration of European laboratories and other resources to respond to requests from actors and agencies in low and middle income countries for specific infectious disease research. In general, most of these approaches favour 'mid-size' networks and infrastructures that are adaptable rather than scaling up to the global level, which can become totalising and inflexible in terms of adaptability to local needs. This aligns with what has been called 'cosmological scalability':

> This approach emphasises diversity, local adaptation, and open knowledge sharing, contrasting with the rigid standardisation and control typical of conventional scaling methods. The concept of cosmolocal production has emerged alongside the proliferation of digital communication networks. It describes methods of connecting local communities through networks of shared resources and knowledge, effectively redefining community in terms of place. This is achieved via infrastructures that facilitate sharing knowledge, techniques, and practices over open communication channels.
>
> *(Kostakis et al 2024, p621)*

Even the goals of downstream patient-centred care and PPIE, which we also advocate, require local flexibilities, adaptation and making space at the level of particular hospitals or even particular clinical encounters to bring the relational, situated aspect of care back in, as a counter to the hegemony of impersonal precision. Even though, ideally, patient-centred care can and should be supported by top-down national policies, it still relies on capacities to act within local networks of healthcare provision to be meaningfully achieved.

Finally, the emphasis on care in this chapter is a reminder that while PM can be beneficial it is never by itself sufficient. Medicine should be informed by data but never determined by it. This is partly an appeal for epistemic humility.

A reminder that the data is always a map, never the territory and should never be taken as the final arbiter of reality. It is also a reminder that medicine is both a scientific *and* a social enterprise and the former cannot be separated from the latter. In the field of artificial intelligence, the need to retain human judgement is often phrased as keeping a 'human in the loop', but more broadly, in data-driven, stratified medicine – whether algorithms are involved or not – we highlight the need to retain the capacity for discretion: to judge when generalised rules should apply to a particular case and when to make a justifiable exemption to account for the messy, relational situatedness of human and more-than-human life (Daston 2023). Thus, our final appeal is to retain a human scale in order to sustain a humane future for PM.

Note

1 Examples of non-excludable goods include the law, natural air, and national defence, among others. A second criterion for qualifying as 'public goods' requires they be non-rival, whereby the use of a good or service by one individual does not prevent others from using it (e.g., natural air).

REFERENCES

23andme. (2024). Your DNA is amazing! *23andme.com.* Available at https://www.23andme.com/en-gb/about/

Abraham, J. (1995). *Science, politics, and the pharmaceutical industry: Controversy and bias in drug regulation.* UCL Press, London.

Adam, B., and Groves, C. (2011). Futures tended: Care and future-oriented responsibility. *Bulletin of Science, Technology and Society, 31*(1): 17–27.

Addison, C. (2017). Spliced: Boundary-work and the establishment of human gene therapy. *BioSocieties, 12*(2): 257–281.

Akrich, M. (1992). De-scription - how technologies are used to attempt to inscribe user behaviours. In W. E. Bijker and J. Law (Eds.), *Shaping technology/building society: Studies in sociotechnical change.* MIT Press, Cambridge: 205–224.

Alkhatib, A. (2021, May). To live in their utopia: Why algorithmic systems create absurd outcomes. *Proceedings of the 2021 CHI conference on human factors in computing systems*, Yokohama, Japan: 1–9.

All of Us. (2023). All of Us: Participation. *National Institutes of Health.* Available at https://allofus.nih.gov/about

Andersen, B., and Arnason, E. (1999). Iceland's database is ethically questionable. *British Medical Journal, 318*(7197): 1565.

Aquino, Y. S. J., Carter, S. M., Houssami, N., Braunack-Mayer, A., Win, K. T., Degeling, C., Wang, L., and Rogers, W. A. (2025). Practical, epistemic and normative implications of algorithmic bias in healthcare artificial intelligence: A qualitative study of multidisciplinary expert perspectives. *Journal of Medical Ethics, 51*(6): 420–428.

Ardizone, G., and Morrison, M. (2026). Engaging with biomodifying therapies: Perspectives of patient group representatives in the UK. *Anthropology and Medicine (forthcoming).*

Arlett, P., Kjær, J., Broich, K., and Cooke, E. (2021). Real-world evidence in EU medicines regulation: Enabling use and establishing value. *Clinical Pharmacology and Therapeutics, 111*(1): 21.

Armstrong, D. (2006). Embodiment and ethics: Constructing medicine's two bodies. *Sociology of Health and Illness, 28*(6): 866–881.

Armstrong, D. (1995). The rise of surveillance medicine. *Sociology of Health and Illness, 17*(3): 393–404.

Article 29 Working Party. (2014). Opinion 05/(2014) on anonymization techniques, October 4. Directive 95/46/EC. Article 29 working party, directorate C (fundamental rights and union citizenship). *European Commission, Directorate General Justice.* Available at https://ec.europa.eu/justice/article-29/documentation/opinion-recommendation/files/(2014)/wp216_en.pdf

Asgarinia, H. (2024). Limiting access to certain anonymous information: From the group right to privacy to the principle of protecting the vulnerable. *The Journal of Value Inquiry*, 1–27. https://doi.org/10.1007/s10790-024-09980-x

Asprey, D. (2017). *Head strong: The bulletproof plan to activate untapped brain energy to work smarter and think faster-in just two weeks (Bulletproof 3).* Harper Wave. Available at https://www.amazon.co.uk/Head-Strong-Bulletproof-Activate-Faster/

Aurucci, P. (2023). *Il trattamento dei dati personali nella ricerca biomedica: Problematiche etico-giuridiche (Prima edizione).* Università degli studi di Torino, Edizioni scientifiche Italiane.

Avior, Y., Sagi, I., and Benvenisty, N. (2016). Pluripotent stem cells in disease modelling and drug discovery. *Nature Reviews Molecular Cell Biology, 17*(3): 170–182.

Azizi, Z., Zheng, C., Mosquera, L., Pilote, L., and El Emam, K. (2021). Can synthetic data be a proxy for real clinical trial data? A validation study. *British Medical Journal Open, 11*(4): e043497.

Baird, A. M., Westphalen, C. B., Blum, S., Nafria, B., Knott, T., Sargeant, I., Harnik, H., Brooke, N., Wicki, N., and Wong-Rieger, D. (2023). How can we deliver on the promise of precision medicine in oncology and beyond? A practical roadmap for action. *Health Science Reports, 6*(6): p.e1349.

Balint, M. (1964). *The doctor, his patient, and the illness.* Pittman Medical, London.

Ballo, R., Pearce, W., Stilgoe, J., and Wilsdon, J. (2024). Socially-distanced science: How British publics were imagined, modelled and marginalised in political and expert responses to the COVID-19 pandemic. *Humanities and Social Sciences Communications, 11*(1): 1–12.

Barry, A. (2006). Technological zones. *European Journal of Social Theory, 9*(2): 239–253.

Barry, A. (2001). *Political machines: Governing a technological society.* Adam and Charles Black Publishers, London.

Bauer, M. W. (2009). The evolution of public understanding of science—discourse and comparative evidence. *Science, Technology and Society, 14*(2): 221–240.

Beer, D. (2016). *Metric power.* Palgrave Macmillan, Basingstoke.

Bellino, S., La Salvia, A., Cometa, M. F., and Botta, R. (2023). Cell-based medicinal products approved in the European Union: Current evidence and perspectives. *Frontiers in Pharmacology, 14*: 1200808.

Berger, I., Ahmad, A., Bansal, A., Kapoor, T., Sipp, D., and Rasko, J. E. (2016). Global distribution of businesses marketing stem cell-based interventions. *Cell Stem Cell, 19*(2): 158–162.

Bianco, P., Barker, R., Brüstle, O., Cattaneo, E., Clevers, H., Daley, G. Q., De Luca, M., Goldstein, L., Lindvall, O., Mummery, C., and Robey, P. G. (2013). Regulation of stem cell therapies under attack in Europe: For whom the bell tolls. *The European Molecular Biology Organization (EMBO) Journal, 32*(11): 1489–1495.

Biasin, E. (2023, September 5). Healthcare AI: Overpromising and under-representative? A legal perspective. *KU Leuven AI Summer School Blog.* Available at https://www.law.kuleuven.be/ai-summer-school/blogpost/Blogposts/AI-healthcare-underrepresentation

Biasin, E., and Kamenjasevic, E. (2022). Cybersecurity of medical devices: Regulatory challenges in the European Union. In C. Shachar, C. Robertson, I. G. Cohen, T. Minssen, and W. N. Price II (Eds.), *The future of medical device regulation: Innovation and protection.* Cambridge University Press, Cambridge: 51–62.

Biasin, E., Kamenjasevic, E., Ludvigsen, K. R., Solaiman, B., and Cohen, I. G. (2023). *Cybersecurity of AI medical devices: Risks, legislation, and challenges.* Cheltenham, UK: Edward Elgar.

Bicudo, E, and Brass, I. (2022). Institutional and infrastructure challenges for hospitals producing advanced therapies in the UK: The concept of point-of-care manufacturing readiness. *Regenerative Medicine, 17*(10): 719–737.

Bicudo, E., Faulkner, A., and Li, P. (2021a). Sociotechnical alignment in biomedicine: The 3D bioprinting market beyond technology convergence. *Technology in Society, 66*: 101668.

Bicudo, E., Faulkner, A., and Li, P. (2021b). Software, risks, and liabilities: Ongoing and emergent issues in 3D bioprinting. *Journal of Risk Research, 24*(10): 1319–1334.

Biomarkers Definition Working Group. (2001). Biomarkers and surrogate endpoints: Preferred definitions and conceptual framework. *Clinical Pharmacology and Therapeutics, 69*: 89–95.

Birch, K. (2017). Rethinking value in the bio-economy: Finance, assetization, and the management of value. *Science, Technology, and Human Values, 42*(3): 460–490.

Blaxter, M. (1978). Diagnosis as category and process: The case of alcoholism, social science and medicine. *Part A: Medical Psychology and Medical Sociology, 12*: 9–17.

Bleher, H., and Braun, M. (2022). Diffused responsibility: Attributions of responsibility in the use of AI-driven clinical decision support systems. *AI and Ethics, 2*(4): 747–761.

Bliss, M. (1983). *The discovery of insulin.* Paul Harris, Edinburgh.

Blood Cancer-UK. (2018). Another CAR-T treatment provisionally turned down for use on NHS. *Blood Cancer UK.* Available at https://bloodcancer.org.uk/news/another-car-t-treatment-provisionally-turned-down-use-nhs/#:~:text=Kymriah%20has%20a%20list%20price,it%20were%20to%20be%20approved

Bontridder, N., Hähnel, T., Valero, M. M., Marín, L. C., Corvol, J. C., El-Yacoubi, M. A., Eskofier, B., Razzouki, A. F., Hansen, A. F., Glaab, E., and Ibrahim, A. A. (2024). Leveraging the potential of digital technology for personalised medicine. *Journal of AI Law and Regulation, 1*(2): 249–253.

Borup, M., Brown, N., Konrad, K., and Van Lente, H. (2006). The sociology of expectations in science and technology. *Technology Analysis and Strategic Management, 18*(3–4): 285–298.

Bourgeron, T., and Geiger, S. (2024). Countermovements from the core: The assetization of pharmaceuticals, transparency activism and the access to medicines movement. *Socio-Economic Review, 22*(4): 1755–1782.

Bowker, G. C. (1994). *Science on the run: Information management and industrial geophysics at Schlumberger, 1920–1940.* MIT Press, Cambridge.

Bowker, G.C., Baker, K., Millerand, F. and Ribes, D. (2010) Toward Information Infrastructure Studies: Ways of Knowing in a Networked Environment. In: Hunsinger, J., Klastrup, L. and Allen, M., Eds., *International Handbook of Internet Research*, Dordrecht: Springer, pp. 97-117. https://doi.org/10.1007/978-1-4020-9789-8_5

Bowker, G. C., and Star, S. L. (1999). *Sorting things out: Classification and its consequences.* (2nd print. eds). MIT Press, Cambridge.

Bradford, L., Aboy, M., and Liddell, K. (2020). COVID-19 contact tracing apps: A stress test for privacy, the GDPR, and data protection regimes. *Journal of Law and the Biosciences, 7*(1): 1–21.

Braun, L., Fausto-Sterling, A., Fullwiley, D., Hammonds, E. M., Nelson, A., Quivers, W., Reverby, S. M., and Shields, A. E. (2007). Racial categories in medical practice: How useful are they? *PLoS medicine, 4*(9): e271.

Briz Hernández, I. (2025). Miscellaneous care: Bridging the in-between of translational medicine. *Science, Technology, and Human Values, 50*(2): 251–273.

Brossard, D., and Lewenstein, B. V. (2009). A critical appraisal of models of public understanding of science: Using practice to inform theory. In L. Kahlor and P. Stout (Eds.), *Communicating science: New agendas in communication.* Routledge, London: 25–53.

Brown, N. (2003). Hope against hype: Accountability in biopasts, presents and futures. *Science Studies, 16*: 3–21.

Brown, N., and Webster, A. (2004). *New medical technologies and society: Reordering life.* Polity Press, Cambridge.

Budin-Ljøsne, I., and Harris, J. R. (2016). Patient and interest organizations' views on personalized medicine: A qualitative study. *BioMed Central (BMC) Medical Ethics, 17*: 1–10.

Businesswire. (2022). European medicines agency qualifies unlearn's AI-powered method for running smaller, faster clinical trials. *Businesswire.com.* Available at https://www.businesswire.com/news/home/20220928005391/en/Europea... n's-AI-powered-Method-for-Running-Smaller-Faster-Clinical-Trials

Butler, J. (1988). Performative acts and gender constitution: An essay in phenomenology and feminist theory. *Theatre Journal, 40*(4): 519–520.

Callon, M., and Rabeharisoa, V. (2008). The growing engagement of emergent concerned groups in political and economic life: Lessons from the French association of neuromuscular disease patients. *Science, Technology, and Human Values, 33*(2): 230–261.

Cambridge Dictionary. (2024). Meaning of 'consumer'. *Cambridge Dictionary.* Available at https://dictionary.cambridge.org/dictionary/english/consumer#google_vignette

Cambrosio, A., Campbell, J., Drilon, A. E., Keating, P., and Polk, J. B. (2024). Decision-making as discovery: Vetting clinical research in a leading precision oncology service. *Sociology of Health and Illness, 46*(3): 495–513.

Cambrosio, A., Keating, P., Vignola-Gagné, E., Besle, S., and Bourret, P. (2018). Extending experimentation: Oncology's fading boundary between research and care. *New Genetics and Society, 37*(3): 207–226.

Canvin, K., Jones, C., Marttila, A., Burström, B., and Whitehead, M. (2007). Can I risk using public services? Perceived consequences of seeking help and health care among households living in poverty: Qualitative study. *Journal of Epidemiology and Community Health, 61*(11): 984–989.

Carter, P., Laurie, G. T., and Dixon-Woods, M. (2015). The social licence for research: Why care. data ran into trouble. *Journal of Medical Ethics, 41*(5): 404–409.

Cave, A., Kurz, X., & Arlett, P. (2019). Real-world data for regulatory decision making: challenges and possible solutions for Europe. *Clinical Pharmacology and Therapeutics, 106*(1), 36–39.

Charatan, F. (2001). US approves new anti-leukaemia drug. *British Medical Journal, 322*: 1201.

Cheng, S., Kerr, K. F., Thiessen-Philbrook, H., Coca, S. G., and Parikh, C. R. (2020). BioPETsurv: Methodology and open source software to evaluate biomarkers for prognostic enrichment of time-to-event clinical trials. *PloS One, 15*(9): e0239486.

Christophersen, M., Mørck, P., Langhoff, T. O., and Bjørn, P. (2015). Unforeseen challenges: Adopting wearable health data tracking devices to reduce health insurance costs in organizations. *Universal access in human-computer interaction. Access to learning, health and well-being: 9th international conference*, UAHCI (2015), Held as Part of HCI International (2015), Los Angeles, CA, August 2–7. Proceedings, Part III 9, Springer International Publishing: 288–299.

CINECA. (n.d.). Common infrastructure for National Cohorts in Europe, Canada, and Africa. Available at https://www.cineca-project.eu/

Clark, P. A., Friedman, J. R., Crosson, D. W., and Fadus, M. (2011). Concierge medicine: Medical, legal and ethical perspectives. *The Internet Journal of Law, Healthcare, and Ethics*, *7*: 1528–8250.

Cole, T. R. (1992). *The journey of life: A cultural history of aging in America*. Cambridge University Press, Cambridge.

Collingridge, D. (1980). *The social control of technology.* St Martin, New York.

Cook, J. A., and Collins, G. S. (2015). The rise of big clinical databases. *Journal of British Surgery, 102*(2): e93–e101.

Crawford, K., Gray, M. L., and Miltner, K. (2014). Big data critiquing big data: Politics, ethics, epistemology. Special section introduction. *International Journal of Communication, 8*: 10.

Cristofaro, L. (2023, October 18). Legal status of synthetic data. *LinkedIn. Com*. Available at https://www.linkedin.com/pulse/legal-status-synthetic-data-lorenzo-cristofaro/

Currie, G. P., Lee, D. K., and Liworth, B. J. (2006). Long-acting β2-agonists in asthma. *Drug Safety, 29*(8): 647–656.

Daily, L. (2019, 22 October). Before you pay extra to join a concierge medical practice, consider these questions. *The Washington Post*. Available at https://www.washingtonpost.com/lifestyle/home/before-you-pay-extra-to-join-a-concierge-medical-practice-consider-these-questions/2019/10/21/90d8206a-ef8b-11e9-b648-76bcf86eb67e_story.html (Accessed: 19 February 2025).

Dam, M. S., Green, S., Bogicevic, I., Hillersdal, L., Spanggaard, I., Rohrberg, K. S., and Svendsen, M. N. (2022). Precision patients: Selection practices and moral pathfinding in experimental oncology. *Sociology of Health and Illness*, *44*(2): 345–359.

Daston, L. (2023, 23 April). The virtue of discretion. *Aeon*. Available at https://aeon.co/essays/discretion-is-hard-to-live-with-even-harder-to-live-without

Daston, L. (1992). Objectivity and the escape from perspective. *Social Studies of Science, 22*(4): 597–618.

Daston, L., and Galison, P. (1992). The image of objectivity. *Representations, 40*: 81–128.

Daston, L., and Galison, P. L. (2021). *Objectivity*. Zone Books, Cambridge.

Datta, S. (2020). Emerging dynamics of evidence and trust in online user-to-user engagement: The case of 'unproven' stem cell therapies. In L. Reynolds and Sariola (Eds.), *The ethics and politics of community engagement in global health research*. Routledge, London: 99–109.

Datta, S. (2018). An endogenous explanation of growth: Direct-to-consumer stem cell therapies in PR China, India and the USA. *Regenerative Medicine, 13*(5): 559–579.

Datta Burton, S., Kieslich, K., Paul, K. T., Samuel, G., and Prainsack, B. (2022). Rethinking value construction in biomedicine and healthcare. *BioSocieties, 17*(3): 391–414.

Datta Burton, S., Mahfoud, T., Aicardi, C., and Rose, N. (2021). Clinical translation of computational brain models: Understanding the salience of trust in clinician–researcher relationships. *Interdisciplinary Science Reviews, 46*(1–2): 138–157.

Davies, G., Frow, E., and Leonelli, S. (2013). Bigger, faster, better? Rhetorics and practices of large-scale research in contemporary bioscience. *BioSocieties, 8*(4): 386–396.

Davis, C., and Abraham, J. (2013). *Unhealthy pharmaceutical regulation: Innovation, politics and promissory science.* Palgrave Macmillan, Basingstoke.

Davis, C., and Abraham, J. (2011). Desperately seeking cancer drugs: Explaining the emergence and outcomes of accelerated pharmaceutical regulation. *Sociology of Health and Illness, 33*: 731–747.

De Saille, S., and Medvecky, F. (2016). Innovation for a steady state: A case for responsible stagnation. *Economy and Society, 45*(1): 1–23.

Delvecchio-Good, M. J. (2001). The biotechnical embrace. *Culture, Medicine and Psychiatry, 25*: 395–410.

Demortain, D. (2017). Expertise, regulatory science and the evaluation of technology and risk: Introduction to the special issue. *Minerva, 55*(2): 139–159.

Demortain, D. (2011). *Scientists and the regulation of risk: Standardising control.* Edward Elgar Publishing, Cheltenham.

Dequech, D. (2001). Bounded rationality, institutions, and uncertainty. *Journal of Economic Issues, 35*(4): 911–929.

Der Standard. (2024, 29 December). 'Krankenkassen-Chef: Dürfen vom Gesundheitssystem nicht Mercedes in Vollausstattung erwarten' (We must not expect the healthcare system to be a well-equipped Mercedes). *Der Standard.* Available at https://www.derstandard.at/story/3000000250977/krankenkassen-chef-duerfen-vom-gesundheitssystem-nicht-mercedes-in-vollausstattung-erwarten

Dewey, J. (1927). *The public and its problems.* Swallow Press Books, Henry Holt and Company, Athens.

Dickenson, D. (2013). *Me medicine vs we medicine: Reclaiming biotechnology for the common good.* Columbia University Press, New York.

DiSalvo, C. (2009). Design and the construction of publics. *Design Issues, 25*(1): 48–63.

Dolan, D. D., Pacia, D. M., Johnston, J., Lee, S. S. J., & Cho, M. K. (2024). Expanding the agenda for a more just genomics. *Hastings Center Report, 54*, S2–S13.

Doerksen, E., Gunay, A. E., Neufeld, S. D., and Friesen, P. (2024). Community-led approaches to research governance: A scoping review of strategies. *Research Ethics*, 21(3), 519–545.

Dolan, D. D., Pacia, D. M., Johnston, J., Lee, S. S. J., and Cho, M. K. (2024). Expanding the agenda for a more just genomics. *Hastings Center Report, 54*: S2–S13.

Douglas, C. M., Aith, F., Boon, W., de Neiva Borba, M., Doganova, L., Grunebaum, S., Hagendijk, R., Lynd, L., Mallard, A., Mohamed, F. A., and Moors, E. (2022). Social pharmaceutical innovation and alternative forms of research, development and deployment for drugs for rare diseases. *Orphanet Journal of Rare Diseases, 17*(1): 344.

Douglas, C. M., and Grunebaum, S. (2024). Lessons learned from the Canadian fabry disease initiative for future risk-sharing and managed access agreements for pharmaceutical and advanced therapies in Canada. *Health Policy, 143*: 105044.

Dove, E. S. (2018). The EU general data protection regulation: Implications for international scientific research in the digital era. *Journal of Law, Medicine and Ethics, 46*(4): 1013–1030.

Dove, E. S., and Özdemir, V. (2015). What role for law, human rights, and bioethics in an age of big data, consortia science, and consortia ethics? The importance of trustworthiness. *Laws, 4*(3): 515.

Dryzek, J. S. (2000). *Deliberative democracy and beyond: Liberals, critics, contestations.* Oxford University Press, Oxford.

Eder, C., and Wild, C. (2019). Technology forecast: Advanced therapies in late clinical research, EMA approval or clinical application via hospital exemption. *Journal of Market Access and Health Policy, 7*(1): 1600939.

EDITH. (2022). European virtual human twin (EDITH). Available at https://www.edith-csa.eu

Edwards, P. N., Jackson, S. J., Bowker, G. C., and Williams, R. (2009). Introduction: An agenda for infrastructure studies. *Journal of the Association for Information Systems, 10*: 364–374.

El Emam, K., Mosquera, L., and Bass, J. (2020). Evaluating identity disclosure risk in fully synthetic health data: Model development and validation. *Journal of Medical Internet Research, 22*(11): e23139.

El-Sayed, S., Kickbusch, I., & Prainsack, B. (2025). Data solidarity: Operationalising public value through a digital tool. *Global Public Health, 20*(1), 2450403.

EP PerMed. (2024). EP PerMed has recently established a citizen engagement board to advise on matters related to citizen engagement in personalised medicine. *European Partnership for Personalised Medicine (EP PerMed) Work Package 5.* Available at https://www.eppermed.eu/news-events/news/ep-permed-citizen-engagement-board-established/#:~:text=Citizen%20engagement%20in%20healthcare%20is,and%20success%20of%20personalised%20medicine.

Epstein, S. (2007). *Inclusion: The politics of difference in medical research.* University of Chicago Press, Chicago.

Epstein, S. (1996). *Impure science: AIDS, activism, and the politics of knowledge* (Vol. 7). University of California Press, Oakland.

Erikainen, S., and Chan, S. (2019). Contested futures: Envisioning "Personalized," "Stratified," and "Precision" medicine. *New Genetics and Society, 38*(3): 308–330.

Eriksson, L. (2016). Pluripotent promises: Configurations of a bio-object. In N. Vermeulen, S. Tamminen, and A. Webster (Eds.), *Bio-objects life in the 21st century.* Routledge, London: 27–42.

Eriksson, L., and Webster, A. (2015). Standardizing work as a recursive process: Shaping the embryonic stem cell field. *New Genetics and Society, 34*(1): 72–88.

Eriksson, L., and Webster, A. (2008). Standardizing the unknown: Practicable pluripotency as doable futures. *Science as Culture, 17*(1): 57–69.

Espeland, W. N. (1997). Authority by the numbers: Porter on quantification, discretion, and the legitimation of expertise. *Law and Social Inquiry, 22*(4): 1107–1133.

EUCAN-Connect. (2019). A federated FAIR platform enabling large-scale analysis of high-value cohort data connecting Europe and Canada in personalized health. *CORDIS-EU.* Available at https://cordis.europa.eu/project/id/824989

European Commission. (2024). European '1+ million genomes' initiative. *European Commission.* Available at https://digital-strategy.ec.europa.eu/en/policies/1-million-genomes

European Commission. (2023). European virtual human twin initiative. *European Commission.* Available at https://digital-strategy.ec.europa.eu/en/policies/virtual-human-twins

European Commission. (2017). International flagship collaboration with Canada for human data storage, integration and sharing to enable personalised medicine approaches. *SC1-BHC-05-2018.* Available at https://ec.europa.eu/info/funding-tenders/opportunities/portal/screen/opportunities/topic-details/sc1-bhc-05-2018

European Court of Justice. (2016). Case C-582/14, Patrick Breyer v Bundesrepublik Deutschland (October 19). *European Court of Justice.* Available at https://curia.europa.eu/juris/document/document. jsf?docid=184668anddoclang=EN

European Data Protection Board. (2021). Guidelines 07/(2020) on the concepts of controller and processor in the GDPR (July 7). *European Data Protection Board.* Available at https://edpb.europa.eu/our-work-tools/our-documents/guidelines/guidelines-072020-concepts-controller-and-processor-gdpr_en

European Data Protection Supervisor. (2015). Mobile health. *European Data Protection Supervisor.* (May 21) Available at https://edps.europa.eu/sites/default/files/publication/15-05-21_mhealth_en_0.pdf

European Data Protection Supervisor. (N.D.). Synthetic data. *European Data Protection Supervisor.* Available at https://edps.europa.eu/press-publications/publications/techsonar/synthetic-data_en

European Medicines Agency. (N.D.). HMA-EMA joint Big Data Steering Group. *European Medicines Agency.* Available at https://www.ema.europa.eu/en/about-us/how-we-work/big-data/hma-ema-joint-big-data-steering-group

European Parliament and of the Council. (2022). Regulation (EU) 2022/868 of the European Parliament and of the council of May 30, 2022, on European data governance and amending regulation (EU) 2018/1724 (Data Governance Act). Available at https://eur-lex.europa.eu/legal-content/EN/TXT/?uri=celex%3A32022R0868

European Science Foundation. (2012). ESF forward look. Personalised medicine for the European citizen. Towards more precise medicine for the diagnosis, treatment and prevention of disease (iPM). *European Science Foundation.* Available at http://archives.esf.org/coordinating-research/forward-looks/biomedical-sciences-med/current-forward-looks-in-biomedical-sciences/personalised-medicine-for-the-european-citizen.html

Faulkner, A. (2012). Tissue engineered technologies: Regulatory pharmaceuticalisation in the European Union. *Innovation: The European Journal of Social Science Research, 25*(4): 389–408.

Faulkner, A. (2009a). Regulatory policy as innovation: Constructing rules of engagement for a technological zone of tissue engineering in the European Union. *Research Policy, 38*: 637–646.

Faulkner, A. (2009b). Chapter 9: Device or drug? Governation of tissue engineering. In A. Faulkner (ed.), *Medical technology into healthcare and society: A sociology of devices, innovation and governance.* Palgrave Macmillan, New York: 159–187.

Faulkner, A. (2009c). *Medical technology into healthcare and society: A sociology of devices, innovation and governance.* Palgrave Macmillan, New York.

Faulkner-Gurstein, R., and Wyatt, D. (2023). Platform NHS: Reconfiguring a public service in the age of digital capitalism. *Science, Technology, and Human Values, 48*(4): 888–908.

Featherstone, K., and Atkinson, P. (2011). *Creating conditions: The making and remaking of a genetic syndrome.* Routledge, London.

Felt, U., Gugglberger, L., and Mager, A. (2009). Shaping the future e-patient. *Science and Technology Studies, 22*: 24–43.

Felt, U., Öchsner, S., and Rae, R. (2020). The making of digital health: Between visions and realizations. Available at https://sts.univie.ac.at/fileadmin/user_upload/i_sts/Publikationen/Projekte/9783830992783-Felt_O__chsner_Rae.pdf

Fenech, M. E., Strukelj, N., and Buston, O. (2018). *Ethical, social, and political challenges of artificial intelligence in health.* Future Advocacy, London.

Ferryman, K., Goldenberg, A. J., and Sabatello, M. (2024). Moving to equity in the All of Us research program. *The American Journal of Bioethics, 24*(3): 115–117.

Finnegan, T., and Hall, A. (2017). *Identification and genomic data.* PHG Foundation, Cambridge.

Fiske, A., Buyx, A., and Prainsack, B. (2019). Health information counsellors: A new profession for the age of big data. *Academic Medicine, 94*(1): 37–41.

Flores, M., Glusman, G., Brogaard, K., Price, N. D., and Hood, L. (2013). P4 medicine: How systems medicine will transform the healthcare sector and society. *Personalized Medicine, 10*(6): 565–576.

Floridi, L. (2014). Open data, data protection, and group privacy. *Philosophy and Technology, 27*: 1–3.

Fontanillo López, C. and A. Elbi. (2022). On synthetic data: a brief introduction for data protection law dummies. Available online at https://europeanlawblog.eu/2022/09/22/on-synthetic-data-a-brief-introduction-for-data-protection-law-dummies/

Forbat, L., Cayless, S., Knighting, K., Cornwell, J., and Kearney, N. (2009). Engaging patients in health care: An empirical study of the role of engagement on attitudes and action. *Patient Education and Counselling, 74*(1): 84–90.

Foucault, M. (1993). About the beginning of the hermeneutics of the self: Two lectures at Dartmouth. Blasius, M. (Ed). *Political Theory, 21*(2): 198–227.

Foucault, M. (1997). The birth of biopolitics. In P. Rabinow (Ed.), *Michel foucault, ethics: Subjectivity and truth.* The New Press, New York: 73–79.

Foucault, M. (1975). *Discipline and Punish.* Translated by Alan Sheridan, Patheon Books, New York.

Foucault, M. (1973). *The birth of the clinic: An archaeology of medical perception.* Tavistock Publications, London.

Freeman, J. L., and Neff, G. (2023). The challenge of repurposed technologies for youth: Understanding the unique affordances of digital self-tracking for adolescents. *New Media and Society, 25*(11): 3047–3064.

Freidlin, B., and Korn, E. (2014). Biomarker enrichment strategies: Matching trial design to biomarker credentials. *Nature Reviews Clinical Oncology, 11*: 81–90.

Gabe, J., and Martin, P. (2023). Chapter 11: Pharmaceuticalisation: Origins, drivers and new developments. In A. Petersen (Ed.), *Handbook on the sociology of health and medicine.* Edward Elgar Publishing Limited, Cheltenham: 170–186.

Galasso, I. (2024). Precision medicine for whom? Public health outputs from "Genomics England" and "All of Us" to make up for upstream and downstream exclusion. *The American Journal of Bioethics, 24*(3): 71–85.

Gardner, J., Faulkner, A., Mahalatchimy, A., and Webster, A. (2015). Are there specific translational challenges in regenerative medicine? Lessons from other fields. *Regenerative Medicine, 10*(7): 885–895.

Gardner, J., and Webster, A. (2016). The social management of biomedical novelty: Facilitating translation in regenerative medicine. *Social Science and Medicine, 156*: 90–97.

Gardner, J., Webster, A., and Barry, J. (2018). Anticipating the clinical adoption of regenerative medicine: Building institutional readiness in the UK. *Regenerative Medicine, 13*(1): 29–39.

Geiger, S., and Gross, N. (2024). Tech sharing, not tech hoarding: Covid-19, global solidarity, and the failed responsibility of the pharmaceutical industry. *Organization, 31*(3): 567–582.

Geiger, S., and Gross, N. (2017). Does hype create irreversibilities? Affective circulation and market investments in digital health. *Marketing Theory, 17*: 435–454.

Geiger, S., and Kjellberg, H. (2021). Market mash ups: The process of combinatorial market innovation. *Journal of Business Research, 124*: 445–457.

Genomic Data Infrastructure. (2022). Genomic Data Infrastructure (GDI). Available at https://gdi.onemilliongenomes.eu

Gilmore, J. H., and Pine, B. J. (1997). The four faces of mass customization. *Harvard Business Review, 75*(1): 91–102.

Gitelman, L., and Jackson, V. (2013). Introduction. In L. Gitelman (Ed.), *Raw data is an oxymoron*. The MIT Press, Cambridge: 1–14. Available at https://direct.mit.edu/books/edited-volume/3992/Raw-Data-Is-an-Oxymoron

Global Alliance for Genomics and Health. (2024). Diversity in datasets policy v2.4. *Global Alliance for Genomics and Health*. Available at https://www.ga4gh.org/document/diversity-in-datasets-policy-v2-4/

GMNation? (2003). GM nation? The findings of the public debate. *History of GM Nation*. Available at www.gmnation.org.uk

GMPublicDebate. (2003). Conduct of the GM public debate. *The UK Parliament. House of Commons. Environment, Food and Rural Affairs Committee*. Available at https://publications.parliament.uk/pa/cm200203/cmselect/cmenvfru/1220/1220.pdf

Goirand, M., Austin, E., and Clay-Williams, R. (2021). Implementing ethics in healthcare AI-based applications: A scoping review. *Science and Engineering Ethics, 27*(5): 61.

Goldberg, C. (2012). Can my company's wellness program really ask me to do that? Available at https://www.wbur.org/news/2012/09/28/wellness-program-legal-limits

Goldenberg, M. J. (2006). On evidence and evidence-based medicine: Lessons from the philosophy of science. *Social Science and Medicine, 62*(11): 2621–2632.

Gonzales, A., Guruswamy, G., and Smith, S. R. (2023). Synthetic data in health care: A narrative review. *PLOS Digital Health, 2*(1): e0000082.

Good Law Project. (N.D.). A win in the fight for transparency over Palantir's NHS data contract. *Good Law Project*. Available at https://goodlawproject.org/update/a-win-in-the-fight-for-transparency-over-palantirs-nhs-data-contract/

Grace, J., and Taylor, M. J. (2013). Disclosure of confidential patient information and the duty to consult: The role of the health and social care information centre. *Medical Law Review, 21*(3): 415–447.

Graf, A. C., Posch, M., and Koenig, F. (2015). Adaptive designs for subpopulation analysis optimizing utility functions. *Biomedical Journal, 57*: 76–89.

Green, S., Carusi, A., and Hoeyer, K. (2022). Plastic diagnostics: The remaking of disease and evidence in personalized medicine. *Social Science and Medicine, 304*: 112318.

Greser, J. (2023, October 17). Synthetic data and medical AI – where do we stand? *LSTS*. Available at https://lsts.research.vub.be/synthetic-data-and-medical-ai-where-do-we-stand

Grisot, M., and Vassilakopoulou, P. (2017). Re-infrastructuring for eHealth: Dealing with turns in infrastructure development. *Computer Supported Cooperative Work (CSCW), 26*(1): 7–31.

Groves, C. (2017). Emptying the future: On the environmental politics of anticipation. *Futures, 92*: 29–38.

Groves, C. (2016). Care and technoscience: Re-embedding the futures of innovation. In D. Bowman, A. Rip, and E. Stokes (Eds.), *Embedding and governing new technologies: A regulatory, ethical and societal perspective*. Jenny Stanford Publishing, Singapore: 89–113.

Groves, C. (2015). Logic of choice or logic of care? Uncertainty, technological mediation and responsible innovation. *Nanoethics, 9*: 321–333.

Gutmann, A., and Thompson, D. (1996). *Democracy and disagreement*. Harvard University Press, Cambridge.

Guttieres, D., Stewart, S., Wolfrum, J., and Springs, S. L. (2019). Cyberbiosecurity in advanced manufacturing models. *Frontiers in Bioengineering and Biotechnology, 7*: 210.

Habermas, J. (1984). *The theory of communicative action (Vol. 2), lifeworld and system: A critique of functionalist reason*. Boston, MA: Beacon Press.

Hacking, I. (2006). Making people up. *London Review of Books*, 28 (16–17): 23–26.

Hall, S. S. (2006). *Size matters: How height affects the health, happiness, and success of boys – and the men they become.* Houghton Mifflin Company, New York.

Hargis, H., and Régnier, F. (2018). Rejecting self-tracking devices: An analysis of refusals of nutrition and fitness apps. *Aliss Notes, 5*: 1–4.

Harris, A., Kelly, S., and Wyatt, S. (2016). *Cybergenetics: Health genetics and new media.* Routledge, Abingdon.

Hauge, A. M. (2024). Regulating diagnosis—Molecular and regulatory sub-stratifications of lung cancer treatment. *Sociology of Health and Illness, 46*(S1): 56–75.

Hauskeller, C., and Weber, S. (2011). Framing pluripotency: iPS cells and the shaping of stem cell science. *New Genetics and Society, 30*(4): 415–431.

Hedgecoe, A. (2004). *The politics of personalised medicine: Pharmacogenetics in the clinic.* Cambridge University Press, Cambridge.

Hedgecoe, A. M. (2003). Terminology and the construction of scientific disciplines: The case of pharmacogenomics. *Science, Technology and Human Values*, *28*(4): 513–537.

Hendrickx, K. (2014). Bodies of evidence: An anthropology of the health claim. Doctoral Thesis, Universite de Liege, Belgium. Available at https://www.researchgate.net/publication/268212591_Bodies_of_Evidence_An_Anthropology_of_the_Health_Claim

Hess, D. J. (2015). Public as threats? Integrating science and technology studies (STS) and social movement studies (SMS). *Science as Culture*, *24*(1): 69–82.

Higdon, R., Haynes, W., Stanberry, L., Stewart, E., Yandl, G., Howard, C., Broomall, W., Kolker, N., and Kolker, E. (2013). Unravelling the complexities of life sciences data. *Big Data, 1*(1): 42–50.

Hilgartner, S. (2015). Capturing the imaginary: Vanguards, visions and the synthetic biology revolution. In S. Hilgartner, C. A. Miller, and R. Hagendijk (Eds.), *Science and democracy*. Routledge, London: 33–55.

Hindorff, L. A., Bonham, V. L., Brody, L. C., Ginoza, M. E., Hutter, C. M., Manolio, T. A., and Green, E. D. (2018). Prioritizing diversity in human genomics research. *Nature Reviews Genetics, 19*(3): 175–185.

Hinterberger, A., and Bea, S. (2023). How do scientists model humanness? A qualitative study of human organoids in biomedical research. *Social Science and Medicine, 320*: 115676.

Hinterberger, A., and Stelmach, A. (2025). Organoids at the forefront of global health: Accelerated research and ethical implications in the cases of Zika and COVID-19. *Global Public Health, 20*(1): 2496679.

Hoeyer, K. (2016). Denmark at a crossroad? Intensified data sourcing in a research radical country. In B. Mittelstadt and L. Floridi (Eds.), *The ethics of biomedical big data. law, governance and technology series*, vol 29. Springer, Cham: 73–93.

Hogle, L. F. (2018). Intersections of technological and regulatory zones in regenerative medicine. In A. Bharadwaj (Ed.), *Global perspectives on stem cell technologies.* Palgrave Macmillan, Cham: 51–84.

Hogle, L. F. (2016). The ethics and politics of infrastructures: Creating the conditions of possibility for big data in medicine. In B. Mittelstadt and L.Floridi (Eds.), *The ethics of biomedical big data. Law, governance and technology series*, vol. 29. Springer, Cham: 397–427.

Hogle, L. F. (2010). Characterizing human embryonic stem cells: Biological and social markers of identity. *Medical Anthropology Quarterly, 24*(4): 433–450.

Hogle, L. F. (2009). Pragmatic objectivity and the standardization of engineered tissues. *Social Studies of Science, 39*(5): 717–742.

Holmberg, T., Schwennesen, N., & Webster, A. (2011). Bio-objects and the bio-objectification process. *Croatian Medical Journal, 52*(6): 740–742.

Horlick-Jones, T., Walls, J., Rowe, G., Pidgeon, N., Poortinga, W., Murdock, G., and O'Riordan, T. (2007). *The GM debate: Risk, politics and public engagement.* Routledge, London.

Horton, R. H., and Lucassen, A. M. (2019). Recent developments in genetic/genomic medicine. *Clinical Science, 133*(5): 697–708.

Hughes, T. P. (1993). *Networks of power: Electrification in Western society, 1880–1930.* Johns Hopkins University Press, Baltimore.

Hutchison, J., and Holdsworth, J. (2021). What choice? Risk and responsibilization in cardiovascular health policy. *Health, 25*(3): 288–305.

ICO. (N.D.). Data Protection Act (1998) undertaking. *Data Controller: Royal Free London NHS Foundation Trust. Ref: RFA0627721.* Available at https://medconfidential.org/wp-content/uploads/2018/05/royal-free-undertaking-03072017.pdf

Ioannidis, J. P. A., and Bossuyt, M. M. (2017). Waste, leaks, and failures in the biomarker pipeline. *Clinical Chemistry, 63*(5): 963–972.

Irwin, A., Jensen, T. E., and Jones, K. E. (2013). The good, the bad and the perfect: Criticizing engagement practice. *Social Studies of Science, 43*(1): 118–135.

Isasi, R., Ginoza, M., Jongsma, K., Assen, L., and Fabbri, M. (2022). Mending the gaps: Ethically sensitive cells and the evolution of European stem cell policy. *Regenerative Medicine, 17*(8): 581–595.

ISIDORe Project. (N.D.). Integrated services for infectious disease outbreak research (ISIDORe). Available at https://isidore-project.eu/

Janiaud, P., Serghiou, S., and Ioannidis, J. P. (2019). New clinical trial designs in the era of precision medicine: An overview of definitions, strengths, weaknesses, and current use in oncology. *Cancer Treatment Reviews, 73*: 20–30.

Jasanoff, S. (2005). *Designs on nature: Science and democracy in Europe and the United States.* Princeton University Press, Princeton.

Jasanoff, S. (2004). *States of knowledge: The co-production of science and the social order.* Routledge, London and New York.

Jasanoff, S., and Kim, S. H. (2015). *Dreamscapes of modernity: Sociotechnical imaginaries and the fabrication of power.* The University of Chicago Press, Chicago.

Jørgensen, J., & Kefalas, P. (2017). Annuity payments can increase patient access to innovative cell and gene therapies under England's net budget impact test. *Journal of Market Access & Health Policy, 5*(1): 1355203.

Jutel, A. (2011). *Putting a name to it: Diagnosis in contemporary society.* Johns Hopkins University Press, Baltimore.

Jutel, A., and Nettleton, S. (2011). Towards a sociology of diagnosis: Reflections and opportunities. *Social Science and Medicine, 73*: 793–800.

Kaba, R., and Sooriakumaran, P. (2007). The evolution of the doctor-patient relationship. *International Journal of Surgery, 5*(1): 57–65.

Kamel Boulos, M. N., and Zhang, P. (2021). Digital twins: From personalised medicine to precision public health. *Journal of Personalized Medicine, 11*(8): 745.

Kammourieh, L., Baar, T., Berens, J., Letouzé, E., Manske, J., Palmer, J., Sangokoya, D., and Vinck, P. (2016). Group privacy in the age of big data. In Linnet Taylor, Luciano Floridi, Bart van der Sloot (eds.), *Group privacy: New challenges of data technologies.* Springer International Publishing, Cham: 37–66.

Kasztura, M., Richard, A., Bempong, N. E., Loncar, D., and Flahault, A. (2019). Cost-effectiveness of precision medicine: A scoping review. *International Journal of Public Health, 64*: 1261–1271.

Kaufman, S. R. (2020). *Ordinary medicine: Extraordinary treatments, longer lives, and where to draw the line*. Duke University Press, Durham.

Kaye, J., Whitley, E. A., Lund, D., Morrison, M., Teare, H., and Melham, K. (2015). Dynamic consent: A patient interface for twenty-first century research networks. *European Journal of Human Genetics, 23*(2): 141–146.

Kelly, S. E. (2009). Choosing not to choose: Reproductive responses of parents of children with genetic conditions or impairments. *Sociology of Health and Illness, 31*: 81–97.

Kemp, P. (2006). History of regenerative medicine: Looking backwards to move forwards. *Regenerative Medicine, 1*(5): 653–669.

Kenny, K., Broom, A., Page, A., Prainsack, B., Wakefield, C. E., Itchins, M., Lwin, Z., and Khasraw, M. (2021). A sociology of precision-in-practice: The affective and temporal complexities of everyday clinical care. *Sociology of Health and Illness, 43*(9): 2178–2195.

Kent, J., Faulkner, A., Geesink, I., & FitzPatrick, D. (2006). Towards governance of human tissue engineered technologies in Europe: Framing the case for a new regulatory regime. *Technological Forecasting and Social Change, 73*(1), 41–60.

Kerasidou, A., and Kerasidou, C. (2023). Data-driven research and healthcare: Public trust, data governance and the NHS. *BioMed Central (BMC) Medical Ethics, 24*(1): 51.

Kerr, A., Hill, R. L., and Till, C. (2018). The limits of responsible innovation: Exploring care, vulnerability and precision medicine. *Technology in Society, 52*: 24–31.

Kerr, A., Key Chekar, C., Ross, E., Swallow, J., and Cunningham-Burley, S. (2021). *Personalised cancer medicine: Future crafting in the genomic era.* Manchester University Press, Manchester.

Khoury, M. J., and Ioannidis, J. P. (2014). Big data meets public health. *Science, 346*(6213): 1054–1055.

Kimmelman, J., and Tannock, I. (2018). The paradox of precision medicine. *Nature Reviews Clinical Oncology, 15*(6): 341–342.

King, S. (2006). Accessing drugs in the eighteenth century regions. In L. Curth (Ed.), *From physick to pharmacology: Five hundred years of British drug retailing*. Ashgate Publishing Limited, Aldershot: 49–78.

Kitchin, R., and McArdle, G. (2016). What makes big data, big data? Exploring the ontological characteristics of 26 datasets. *Big Data and Society, 3*(1): 2053951716631130.

Kleinhout-Vliek, T. H., Boon, W. P. C., Hagendijk, R. P., Hoekman, J., and Moors, E. H. M. (2024). Together for the greater goods: Legitimising social innovation in the pharmaceutical field. *Innovation: The European Journal of Social Science Research, 37*(1): 60–84.

Kohlberger, T., and Liu, Y. (2020, February 19). Generating diverse synthetic medical image data for training machine learning models. *Google AI Blog*. Available at https://research.google/blog/generating-diverse-synthetic-medical-image-data-for-training-machine-learning-models/

Kokott, J., and Sobotta, C. (2013). The distinction between privacy and data protection in the jurisprudence of the CJEU and the ECTHR. *International Data Privacy Law, 3*(4): 222–228.

Kostakis, V., Lemos, L., and Kouvara, A. (2024). Another scalability is possible! From non-scalability to cosmolocal scalability. TripleC: Communication, capitalism and critique. *Open Access Journal for a Global Sustainable Information Society, 22*(2): 620–629.

Kraft, S. A., Cho, M. K., Gillespie, K., Halley, M., Varsava, N., Ormond, K. E., Luft, H. S., Wilfond, B. S., and Lee, S. S.-J. (2018). Beyond consent: Building trusting relationships with diverse populations in precision medicine research. *The American Journal of Bio ethics, 18*(4): 3–20.

Krankenkassen-Chef: "Dürfen vom Gesundheitssystem nicht Mercedes in Vollausstattung erwarten"'. Der Standard (29 December 2024), Available at: https://www.derstandard.at/story/3000000250977/krankenkassen-chef-duerfen-vom-gesundheitssystem-nicht-mercedes-in-vollausstattung-erwarten (accessed 24 February 2026)

Krisam, J., and Kieser, M. (2015). Performance of biomarker-based subgroup selection rules in adaptive enrichment designs. *Statistical Biosciences, 8*: 8–27.

Krisam, J., and Kieser, M. (2014). Decision rules for subgroup selection based on a predictive biomarker. *Journal of Biopharmaceutical Statistics, 24*: 188–202.

Kuch, D., Kearnes, M., and Gulson, K. (2020). The promise of precision: Datafication in medicine, agriculture and education. *Policy Studies, 41*(5): 527–546.

Lanar, S., Acquadro, C., Seaton, J., Savre, I., and Arnould, B. (2020). To what degree are orphan drugs patient-centered? A review of the current state of clinical research in rare diseases. *Orphanet Journal of Rare Diseases, 15*(1): 134.

Landecker, H. (2007). *Culturing life: How cells became technologies.* Harvard University Press, Cambridge.

Landry, L. G., Ali, N., Williams, D. R., Rehm, H. L., and Bonham, V. L. (2018). Lack of diversity in genomic databases is a barrier to translating precision medicine research into practice. *Health Affairs, 37*(5): 780–785.

Larkin, B. (2013). The politics and poetics of infrastructure. *Annual Review of Anthropology, 42*(1): 327–343.

Latimer, J., Featherstone, K., Atkinson, P., Clarke, A., Pilz, D. T., and Shaw, A. (2006). Rebirthing the clinic: The interaction of clinical judgment and genetic technology in the production of medical science. *Science, Technology, and Human Values, 31*(5): 599–630.

Latour, B., Salk, J., and Woolgar, S. (1986). *Laboratory life: The construction of scientific facts.* Princeton University Press, Princeton.

Law, J. (1987). Technology, closure and heterogeneous engineering: The case of the Portuguese expansion. In W. E. Bijker, T. P. Hughes, and T. J. Pinch (Eds.), *The social construction of technological systems, new directions in the sociology and history of technology*. MIT Press, Cambridge: 105–128.

Lawler, M., and Sullivan, R. (2015). Personalised and precision medicine in cancer clinical trials: Panacea for progress or Pandora's box? *Public Health Genomics, 18*: 329–337.

Lay, W., Gasparini, L., Siero, W., and Hughes, E. K. (2024). A rapid review of the benefits and challenges of dynamic consent. *Research Ethics21*(1), 180–202.

Ledford, H. (2019). Millions of black people affected by racial bias in health-care algorithms. *Nature, 574*: 608–609.

Lee, J. A., Cho, A., Huang, E. N., Xu, Y., Quach, H., Hu, J., and Wong, A. P. (2021). Gene therapy for cystic fibrosis: New tools for precision medicine. *Journal of Translational Medicine, 19*: 1–15.

Lee, J. M., and Howell, J. D. (2006). Tall girls: The social shaping of a medical therapy. *Archives of Pediatric and Adolescent Medicine, 60*: 1035–1039.

Lee, J. Y. (2023). Personalising social ills: An analysis of race-based genomics and personalised medicine. *Journal of Law and Medicine*, *30*(4), 884–898.

Lemke, T. (2010). *Biopolitics: An advanced introduction.* New York University Press, New York.

Lemke, T. (2001). 'The birth of bio-politics': Michel Foucault's lecture at the Collège de France on neo-liberal governmentality. *Economy and Society, 30*(2): 190–207.

Lester, D. S. (2009). Will personalized medicine help in 'transforming' the business of healthcare? *Personalized Medicine, 6*(5): 555–565.

Lezaun, J. & Soneryd, L. (2006) Government by elicitation: engaging stakeholders or listening to the idiots? Discussion Paper 34, Centre for Analysis of Risk and Regulation, London School of Economics. http://www.lse.ac.uk/collections/CARR/pdf/DPs/Disspaper34.pdf

Li, P., Faulkner, A., and Medcalf, N. (2020). 3D bioprinting in a 2D regulatory landscape: Gaps, uncertainties, and problems. *Law, Innovation and Technology*, *12*(1): 1–29.

Lievevrouw, E. (2023). 'Moving focus'. Understanding the infrastructuring of digital health technologies through EU and US policymaking. Available at https://lirias.kuleuven.be/3978594

Lievevrouw, E., and Felt, U. (2026). Governing citizen-patients: The digital infrastructuring of health and care in Europe. In B. Marent (Ed.), *De Gruyter handbook of digital health and society*. Berlin: De Gruyter, pp. 255–278.

Lievevrouw, E., Marelli, L., and Van Hoyweghen, I. (2024). Weaving EU digital health policy into national healthcare practices. The making of a reimbursement standard for digital health technologies in Belgium. *Social Science and Medicine*, *346*: 116620.

Lievevrouw, E., Marelli, L., and Van Hoyweghen, I. (2021). The FDA's standard-making process for medical digital health technologies: Co-producing technological and organizational innovation. *Biosocieties, 17*(3): 549.

Lindfors, A. (2024). Between self-tracking and alternative medicine: Biomimetic imaginary in contemporary biohacking. *Body and Society, 30*(1): 83–110.

Lindpaintner, K. (2004). The role of genotyping in pharmacological therapy. In M. R. Wilkins and E. D. Abel (Eds.), *Cardiovascular pharmacogenetics.* Springer Verlag, New York: 1–24.

Liu, Z., Chen, J., Wang, K., Wang, B., and Zhang, C. (2021). Current status and opportunities in adaptive data analysis for therapeutic cell manufacturing. *Current Opinion in Biomedical Engineering, 20*: 100351.

Livingstone, D. N. (2003). *Putting science in its place: Geographies of scientific knowledge.* Chicago University Press, Chicago.

Lupton, D. (2003). The body in medicine. In D. Lupton (Ed.), *Medicine as culture: Illness, disease and the body in western societies* (2nd edition). Sage, London: 20–49.

Lysaght, T., Lipworth, W., Hendl, T., Kerridge, I., Lee, T. L., Munsie, M., Waldby, C., and Stewart, C. (2017). The deadly business of an unregulated global stem cell industry. *Journal of Medical Ethics, 43*(11): 744–746.

Macaskill, E., and Dance, G. (2013). NSA files. Decoded. What the revelations mean for you. *The Guardian.* Available at https://www.theguardian.com/world/interactive/2013/nov/01/snowden-nsa-files-surveillance-revelations-decoded

Mager, A., and Katzenbach, C. (2021). Future imaginaries in the making and governing of digital technology: Multiple, contested, commodified. *New Media and Society, 23*(2): 223–236.

Mahnke, C. B. (2000). The growth and development of a specialty: The history of pediatrics. *Clinical Pediatrics, 39*(12): 705–714.

Mantelero, A. (2016). Personal data for decisional purposes in the age of analytics: From an individual to a collective dimension of data protection. *Computer Law and Security Review, 32*(2): 238–255.

Mantle, J. L., Rammohan, J., Romantseva, E. F., Welch, J. T., Kauffman, L. R., McCarthy, J., Schiel, J., Baker, J. C., Strychalski, E. A., Rogers, K. C., and Lee, K. H. (2019). Cyberbiosecurity for biopharmaceutical products. *Frontiers in Bioengineering and Biotechnology, 7*: 116.

Martin, P. (1999). Genes as drugs: The social shaping of gene therapy and the reconstruction of genetic disease. *Sociology of Health and Illness, 21*(5): 517–538.

Martin, P., Morrison, M., Turkmendag, I., Nerlich, B., McMahon, A., De Saille, S., and Bartlett, A. (2020). Genome editing: The dynamics of continuity, convergence, and change in the engineering of life. *New Genetics and Society, 39*(2): 219–242.

Martin, P. A., Coveney, C., Kraft, A., Brown, N., and Bath, P. (2006). Commercial development of stem cell technology: Lessons from the past, strategies for the future. *Regenerative Medicine, 1*(6): 801–807.

Mason, C. (2007). Regenerative medicine 2.0. *Regenerative Medicine, 2*(1): 11–18.

McCall, C. (2018). Opt-out digital health records cause debate in Australia. The *Lancet, 392*(10145): 372.

McFall, L. (2019). Personalizing solidarity? The role of self-tracking in health insurance pricing. *Economy and Society, 48*(1): 52–76.

McFall, L., Meyers, G., and Hoyweghen, I. V. (2020). The personalisation of insurance: Data, behaviour and innovation. *Big Data and Society, 7*(2): 2053951720973707.

McLean, A. K., Stewart, C., and Kerridge, I. (2015). Untested, unproven, and unethical: The promotion and provision of autologous stem cell therapies in Australia. *Stem Cell Research and Therapy, 6*(1): 33.

McMahon, A. (2021). Global equitable access to vaccines, medicines and diagnostics for COVID-19: The role of patents as private governance. *Journal of Medical Ethics, 47*(3): 142–148.

McShane, L. M., Rothmann, M. D., and Fleming, T. R. (2023). Finding the (biomarker-defined) subgroup of patients who benefit from a novel therapy: No time for a game of hide and seek. *Clinical Trials, 20*(4): 341–350.

McWhinney I. (1989). The need for a transformed clinical method. In M. Stewart and D. Roter (Eds.), *Communicating with medical patients*. Sage, London: 25–40.

Medvei, V. C. (1993). *The history of clinical endocrinology: A comprehensive account of endocrinology from earliest times to the present day.* The Parthenon Publishing Group Limited, Carnforth.

Mehta, C., Schäfer, H., Daniel, H., and Irle, S. (2014). Biomarker driven population enrichment for adaptive oncology trials with time to event endpoints. *Statistics in Medicine, 33*(26): 4515–4531.

Merriam-Webster. (2024). Definition of 'patient'. Available at https://www.merriam-webster.com/dictionary/patient

Meseguer-Ripolles, J., Khetani, S. R., Blanco, J. G., Iredale, M., and Hay, D. C. (2018). Pluripotent stem cell-derived human tissue: Platforms to evaluate drug metabolism and safety. *The American Association of Pharmaceutical Scientists (AAPS) Journal, 20*: 1–10.

Meskus, M. (2018). *Craft in biomedical research: The iPS cell technology and the future of stem cell science.* Palgrave Macmillan, Basingstoke.

Meszaros, J., Ho, C., and Corrales Compagnucci, M. (2020). Nudging consent and the new opt-out system to the processing of health data in England. In M. C. Compagnucci, N. Forgó, T. Kono, S. Teramoto, and E. P. M. Vermeulen (Eds.), *Legal tech and the new sharing economy.* Springer, Singapore: 93–113.

Meyers, G. (2018). Behaviour-based personalisation in health insurance: A sociology of a not-yet market. Doctoral Thesis, KU Leuven, Belgium. Available at https://kuleuven.limo.libis.be/discovery/search?query=any,contains,LIRIAS2087689andtab=LIRIASandsearch_scope=lirias_profileandvid=32KUL_KUL:Liriasandoffset=0

Michael, M. (1998). Between citizen and consumer: Multiplying the meanings of the "public understanding of science". *Public Understanding of Science, 7*: 313–327.

Miller, B. (2021). Is technology value-neutral? *Science, Technology, and Human Values, 46*(1): 53–80.

Miller, G., Kuch, D., and Kearnes, M. (2022). Reimagining health as a 'flow on effect' of biomedical innovation: Research policy as a site of state activism. *Minerva, 60*(2): 235–256.

Milmo, D. (2021). Frances Haugen to testify to MPs about Facebook and online harm. *The Guardian.* Available at https://www.theguardian.com/technology/2021/oct/25/frances-haugen-to-testify-to-mps-about-facebook-and-online-harm

Minari, J., Brothers, K. B., and Morrison, M. (2018). Tensions in ethics and policy created by National Precision Medicine Programs. *Human Genomics, 12*(1): 22.

Mittra, J. (2013). Repairing the 'Broken Middle'of the Health Innovation Pathway: Exploring Diverse Practitioner Perspectives on the Emergence and Role of 'Translational Medicine'. *Science & Technology Studies, 26*(3), 103–123.

Modi, N. D., Kichenadasse, G., Hoffmann, T. C., Haseloff, M., Logan, J. M., Veroniki, A. A., Venchiarutti, R. L., Smit, A. K., Tuffaha, H., Jayasekara, H., Manning-Bennet, A., Morton, E., McKinnon, R. A., Rowland, A., Sorich, M. J., and Hopkins, A. M. (2023). A 10-year update to the principles for clinical trial data sharing by pharmaceutical companies: Perspectives based on a decade of literature and policies. *BioMed Central (BMC) Medicine, 21*(1): 400.

Mol, A. (1999). Ontological politics: A word and some questions. *The Sociological Review, 47*: 74–89.

Moreira, T. (2015). Understanding the role of patient organizations in health technology assessment. *Health Expectations, 18*(6): 3349–3357.

Morley, J., Machado, C. C., Burr, C., Cowls, J., Joshi, I., Taddeo, M., and Floridi, L. (2020). The ethics of AI in health care: A mapping review. *Social Science and Medicine, 260*: 113172.

Morley, J. E. (2004). A brief history of geriatrics. *Journals of Gerontology Series A-Biological Sciences and Medical Sciences, 59*(11): 1132–1152.

Morrison, M. (2019). Making cells worthwhile: Calculations of value in a European consortium for induced pluripotent stem cells banking. *Science as Culture, 28*(1): 46–69.

Morrison, M. (2017). Infrastructural expectations: Exploring the promise of international large-scale pluripotent stem cell banks. *New Genetics and Society, 36*(1): 66–83.

Morrison, M. (2015). Growth hormone, enhancement and the pharmaceuticalisation of short stature. *Social Science and Medicine, 131*: 305–312.

Morrison, M. (2012). Promissory futures and possible pasts: The dynamics of contemporary expectations in regenerative medicine. *Biosocieties, 7*: 3–22.

Morrison, M., and Kelly, S. E. (2021). Chapter 9: Personalised medicine. In K. Chamberlain and A. Lyons (Eds.), *Routledge international handbook of critical issues in health and illness.* Routledge, London: 95–107.

Morrison, M., Teare, H., Bertier, G., Buchanan, J., Bylstra, Y., Gaff, C., Jackson, L., Kato, K., Kaufmann, E., Kelly, S., and Lázaro-Muñoz, G. (2020). Implications of secondary findings for clinical contexts. In M. Langanke, P. Erdmann, and K. B. Brothers (Eds.), *Secondary findings in genomic research.* Academic Press, London: 155–201.

Mourby, M., Mackey, E., Elliot, M., Gowans, H., Wallace, S. E., Bell, J., Smith, H., Aidinlis, S., and Kaye, J. (2018). Are 'pseudonymised' data always personal data? Implications of the GDPR for administrative data research in the UK. *Computer Law and Security Review, 34*(2): 222–233.

Mourby, M., and Molnar-Gabor, F. (2025). Chapter 5: Secondary uses of patients' data in the European health data space: A UK-German comparison. In E. S. Dove (Ed.), *Confidentiality, privacy, and data protection in biomedicine.* Routledge, London: 127–149.

Murali, N., and Kogut-Czarkowska, M. (2024, 25 January). Synthetic data—A miracle cure or a data protection headache? *Timelex Blog*. Available at https://www.timelex.eu/en/blog/synthetic-data-miracle-cure-or-data-protection-headache

Mykhalovskiy, E., and Weir, L. (2004). The problem of evidence-based medicine: Directions for social science. *Social Science and Medicine, 59*(5): 1059–1069.

Nedelsky, J. (1990). Law, boundaries and the bounded self. *Representations, 30*: 162–189.

Nelkin, D., and Lindee, M. S. (1995). *The DNA mystique: The gene as a cultural icon*. Freeman, New York.

Nelson, N. C., Keating, P., and Cambrosio, A. (2013). On being "actionable": Clinical sequencing and the emerging contours of a regime of genomic medicine in oncology. *New Genetics and Society, 32*: 405–428.

Nguyen, H. (2024). Americans embrace self-monitoring: A look at app-based health tracking habits. Available at https://yougov.com/en-us/articles/49119-americans-health-tracking-habits-2024s

NHS. (n.d.). More ways to kickstart your health. *National Health Service*. Available at https://www.nhs.uk/better-health/

NHS England. (2024). Privacy Impact Assessment: Care.data. *National Health Service England*. Available at https://www.england.nhs.uk/wp-content/uploads/2014/04/cd-pia.pdf

NHS England. (2018). National data opt-out: Factsheet 5 – setting a national data opt-out. *National Health Service England*. Available at https://www.cfpdrsbhattandszyszko.nhs.uk/wp-content/uploads/2023/04/National-data-Opt-Out.pdf

NICE. (2016). *Community engagement: Improving health and wellbeing and reducing health inequalities*. National Institute for Care and Health Excellence, London. Available at https://www.nice.org.uk/guidance/ng44

NICE. (2008). *Community engagement for health and wellbeing*. National Institute for Care and Health Excellence, London.

Nielsen, J., Kaldor, J., Irwin, A., Stewart, C., and Nicol, D. (2021). Bespoke regulation for bespoke medicine? A comparative analysis of bioprinting regulation in Europe, the USA and Australia. *Journal of 3D Printing in Medicine, 5*(3): 155–167.

NIH Pragmatic Trials Collabratory. (N.D.). Acquiring real-world data. Section 2: Common real-world data sources. *National Institutes of Health (NIH) Pragmatic Trials Collabratory*. Available at https://rethinkingclinicaltrials.org/chapters/conduct/acquiring-real-world-data/common-real-world-data-sources/

Nimmesgern, E., Norstedt, I., and Draghia-Akli, R. (2017). Enabling personalized medicine in Europe by the European Commission's funding activities. *Personalised Medicine, 14*: 355–365.

Nordfalk, F., and Hoeyer, K. (2020). The rise and fall of an opt-out system. *Scandinavian Journal of Public Health, 48*(4): 400–404.

Obermeyer, Z., Powers, B., Vogeli, C., and Mullainathan, S. (2019). Dissecting racial bias in an algorithm used to manage the health of populations. *Science, 336*: 447–453.

Oborn, E., and Barrett, S. (2016). Digital health and citizen engagement: Changing the face of health service delivery. *Health Services Management Research, 29*(1–2): 16–20.

Ocloo, J., and Matthews, R. (2016). From tokenism to empowerment: Progressing patient and public involvement in healthcare improvement. *British Medical Journal (BMJ) Quality and Safety, 25*(8): 626–632.

Ohm, P. (2010). Broken promises of privacy: Responding to the surprising failure of anonymization. *UCLA Law Review, 57*: 1701.

Ohno-Machado, L. (2013). Health surveillance using the internet and other sources of information. *Journal of the American Medical Informatics Association, 20*(3): 403.

Ohno-Machado, L. (2012). Big science, big data, and a big role for biomedical informatics. *Journal of the American Medical Informatics Association, 19*(e1): e1.

Osunsami, S. (2013). *CVS Pharmacy wants workers' health information, or they'll pay a fine*. Available at https://abcnews.go.com/blogs/health/2013/03/20/cvs-pharmacy-wants-workers-health-information-or-theyll-pay-a-fine

Oudshoorn, N. (1994). *Beyond the natural body: An archaeology of sex hormones*. Routledge, London.

Oxford English Dictionary. (N.D.). Infrastructure. Oxford English Dictionary. Available online at https://www.oxfordlearnersdictionaries.com/definition/english/infrastructure

Panofsky, A., and Donovan, J. (2019). Genetic ancestry testing among white nationalists: From identity repair to citizen science. *Social Studies of Science, 49*(5): 653–681.

Parens, E. (Ed.) (2006). *Surgically shaping children: Technology, ethics and the pursuit of normality.* The Johns Hopkins University Press, Baltimore.

Partner MD (2025). Concierge medicine: Costs, factors, and considerations. Available at https://www.partnermd.com/blog/concierge-medicine-costs-factors-considerations

Perez, C. C. (2019). *Invisible women: Data bias in a world designed for men.* Chatto and Windus, London.

Petersen, A., Munsie, M., Tanner, C., MacGregor, C., and Brophy, J. (2017). *Stem cell tourism and the political economy of hope.* Palgrave Macmillan, London.

Petersen, A., Schermuly, A. C., and Anderson, A. (2019). The shifting politics of patient activism: From bio-sociality to bio-digital citizenship. *Health, 23*(4): 478–494.

Petsophonsakul, P., Pirmani, A., De Brouwer, E., Akand, M., Botermans, W., Van Der Aa, F., Vermeesch, J. R., Offner, F., Wuyts, R., Moreau, Y., Maes, I., Blockx, I., Van Rompuy, P., Lewi, M., and Vannieuwenhuyse, B. (2022). Augmenting therapeutic effectiveness through novel analytics (Athena): A public and private partnership project funded by the Flemish government (VLAIO). In B. Séroussi, P. Weber, F. Dhombres, C. Grouin, J.-D. Liebe, S. Pelayo, A. Pinna, B. Rance, L. Sacchi, A. Ugon, A. Benis, and P. Gallos (Eds.), *Studies in Health Technology and Informatics.* IOS Press, pp. 829–833.

Petts, J. (1995). Waste management strategy development: A case study of community involvement and consensus-building in Hampshire. *Journal of Environmental Planning and Management, 38*(4): 519–536.

Pichl, A. (2019). What keeps an outdated stem cell concept alive? A search for traces in science and society. In C. Hauskeller, A. Manzeschke, and A. Pichl (Eds.), *The matrix of stem cell research: An approach to rethinking science in society.* Routledge, London: 131–148.

Pinch, T. (1993). "Testing-One, Two, Three... Testing!" Toward a sociology of testing. *Science, Technology, and Human Values, 18*(1): 25–41.

Pinch, T. J., & Bijker, W. E. (1984). The social construction of facts and artefacts: Or how the sociology of science and the sociology of technology might benefit each other. *Social Studies of Science*, *14*(3), 399–441.

Pinches, E. (2024). CAR-T therapy, Kymriah, available routinely on NHS for form of childhood and young-adult leukaemia. *Blood Cancer UK.* Available at https://bloodcancer.org.uk/news/car-t-therapy-kymriah-available-routinely-on-nhs-for-form-of-childhood-and-young-adult-leukaemia/

Pipek, V., and Wulf, V. (2009). Infrastructuring: Toward an integrated perspective on the design and use of information technology. *Journal of the Association for Information Systems*, *10*: 447–473.

Poell, T., Nieborg, D., & van Dijck, J. (2019). Platformisation. *Internet Policy Review*, *8*(4): 1–13.

Polk, J. B., Campbell, J., Drilon, A., Keating, P., and Cambrosio, A. (2023). Organizing precision medicine: A case study of Memorial Sloan Kettering Cancer Center's engagement in/with genomics. *Social Science and Medicine, 324*: 115789.

Porter, T. M. (1995). *Trust in numbers: The Pursuit of objectivity in science and public life.* Princeton University Press, Princeton.

Powles, J., and Hodson, H. (2017). Google DeepMind and healthcare in an age of algorithms. *Health and Technology, 7*(4): 351–367.

Powell, A. B., Ustek-Spilda, F., Lehuedé, S., & Shklovski, I. (2022). Addressing ethical gaps in 'Technology for Good': Foregrounding care and capabilities. *Big Data & Society, 9*(2), 20539517221113774.

Prainsack, B. (2022). The advent of automated medicine? The values and meanings of precision. In M. Barilan, M. Brusa, and A. Ciechanover (Eds.), *Can precision medicine be personal; can personalised medicine be precise?* Oxford University Press, Oxford: 203–216.

Prainsack, B. (2020). The meaning and enactment of openness in personalised and precision medicine. *Science and Public Policy, 47*(5): 647–654.

Prainsack, B. (2017a). *Personalized medicine: Empowered patients in the 21st century?* New York University Press, New York.

Prainsack, B. (2017b). The "we" in the "me" solidarity and health care in the era of personalized medicine. *Science, Technology, and Human Values, 43*(1): 21–44.

Prainsack, B. (2014). The powers of participatory medicine. *PLoS Biology, 12*(4): 1–2.

Prainsack, B., and Kickbusch, I. (2024). A new public health approach to data: Why we need data solidarity. *British Medical Journal,* 386, q2076.

Precision Medicine Initiative (PMI) Working Group Report to the Advisory Committee to the Director, NIH. (2015). The precision medicine initiative cohort program – building a research foundation for 21st century medicine. Available at https://apo.org.au/node/196181

Presser, L., Hruskova, M., Rowbottom, H., and Kancir, J. (2015). Care data and access to UK health records: Patient privacy and public trust. *Technology Science, 2015081103*: 1–35.

Rabeharisoa, V., and Bourret, P. (2009). Staging and weighting evidence in biomedicine: Comparing clinical practices in cancer genetics and psychiatric genetics. *Social Studies of Science, 39*: 691–715.

Rabeharisoa, V., Moreira, T., and Akrich, M. (2014). Evidence-based activism: Patients', users' and activists' groups in knowledge society. *BioSocieties, 9*(2): 111–128.

Radin, M. J. (1996). *Contested commodities. The trouble with trade in sex, children, body parts, and other things.* Harvard University Press, Cambridge.

Ravetz, J. R. (1987). Usable knowledge, usable ignorance. Incomplete science with policy implications. *Knowledge: Creation, Diffusion, Utilization, 9*(1): 87–116.

Reardon, J. (2017). *The postgenomic condition: Ethics, justice and knowledge after the genome*. The University of Chicago Press, Chicago.

Regalado, A. (2021, April 13). Biotechnology and health: This family raised millions to get experimental gene therapy for their children. *MIT Technology Review*. Available at https://www.technologyreview.com/2021/04/13/1022210/gene-therapy-expensive-treatment-genetic-diseases/

Reimann, M., Eppinger, E., Kamprath, M., and Braun, A. (2012). Beyond the blockbuster model? Personalised medicine as driver for new business models in the pharmaceutical industry. In *Proceedings of the RandD management conference: Value creation and value capture.* Grenoble: 23–25. Available at https://papers.ssrn.com/sol3/papers.cfm?abstract_id=2156976

Reinhardt, U. E. (2002). "Boutique medicine" in the US: Doctors are more interested in having high incomes than providing better health care. *British Medical Journal, 324*(7349): 1335.

Reiser, S. J. (1993). The era of the patient - Using the experience of illness in shaping the missions of health-care. *Journal of the American Medical Association, 269*(8): 1012–1017.

Rheinberger, H.-J. (1997). *Toward a history of epistemic things: Synthesizing proteins in the test tube.* Stanford University Press, Stanford.

Rose, N. (1999). *Powers of freedom: Reframing political thought.* Cambridge University Press, Cambridge.

Rose, N., and Novas, C. (2005). Biological citizenship. In A. Ong and S. Collier (Eds.), *Global assemblages: Technology, politics and ethics as anthropological problems.* Blackwell Publishing, Malden: 439–463.

Rosemann, A. (2019). Alter-standardizing clinical trials: The gold standard in the crossfire. *Science as Culture, 28*(2): 125–148.

Rosemann, A., Bortz, G., Vasen, F., and Sleeboom-Faulkner, M. (2016). Global regulatory developments for clinical stem cell research: Diversification and challenges to collaborations. *Regenerative Medicine, 11*(7): 647–657.

Rosenberg, C. E. (1992). Introduction: Framing disease: Illness, society and history. In C. E. Rosenberg and J. L. Golden (Eds.), *Framing disease: Studies in cultural history.* Rutgers University Press, New Brunswick: xiii–xxvi.

Rothstein, M. A. (2024). Do medically underserved individuals benefit from participating in all of us? *The American Journal of Bioethics, 24*(3): 94–96.

Rothstein, M. A. (2017). Structural challenges of precision medicine: Currents in contemporary bioethics. *The Journal of Law, Medicine and Ethics, 45*(2): 274–279.

Rowley, E., and Martin, P. (2009). *Barriers to commercialisation and utilisation of regenerative medicine in the UK.* Institute for Science and Society, University of Nottingham, Nottingham.

Rubin, D. B. (1993). Statistical disclosure limitation. *Journal of Official Statistics, 2*(2): 461–498.

Saesen, R., Van Hemelrijck, M., Bogaerts, J., Booth, C. M., Cornelissen, J. J., Dekker, A., Eisenhauer, E. A., Freitas, A., Gronchi, A., Hernán, M. A., and Hulstaert, F. (2023). Defining the role of real-world data in cancer clinical research: The position of the european organisation for research and treatment of cancer. *European Journal of Cancer, 186*: 52–61.

Salter, B., and Faulkner, A. (2011). State strategies of governance in biomedical innovation: Aligning conceptual approaches for understanding "Rising Powers" in the global context. *Globalization and Health, 7*: 1–14.

Salter, B., Zhou, Y., and Datta, S. (2017). Governing new global health-care markets: The case of stem cell treatments. *New Political Economy, 22*(1): 76–91.

Salter, B., Zhou, Y., and Datta, S. (2014). Health consumers and stem cell therapy innovation: Markets, models and regulation. *Regenerative Medicine, 9*(3): 353–366.

Samuel, G., & Lucassen, A. M. (2022). The environmental sustainability of data-driven health research: A scoping review. *Digital Health, 8*, 20552076221111297.

Satariano, A. (2014). Wear this device so the boss knows you're losing weight. *Bloomberg.com.* Available at https://www.bloomberg.com/news/articles/2014-08-21/wear-this-device-so-the-boss-knows-you-re-losing-weight?embedded-checkout=true

Sayer, A. (2011). *Why things matter to people: Social science, values and ethical life.* Cambridge University Press, Cambridge.

Schraer, R. (2021, 15 February). Covid-19: Vaccine as good in 'real world' as in trial in Israel. Available at https://www.bbc.co.uk/news/health-56069460

Scott, J. C. (1998). *Seeing like a state: How certain schemes to improve the human condition have failed.* Yale University Press, New Haven.

Selin, C., and Guimarães Pereira, Â. (2013). Pursuing plausibility. *International Journal of Foresight and Innovation Policy, 9*(2–4): 93–109.

Sethi, N. (2019). Regulating for uncertainty: bridging blurred boundaries in medical innovation, research and treatment. *Law, Innovation and Technology, 11*(1), 112–133.

Sharon, T. (2017). Self-tracking for health and the quantified self: Re-articulating autonomy, solidarity, and authenticity in an age of personalized healthcare. *Philosophy of Technology, 30*: 93–121.

Sharp, L. A. (2000). The commodification of the body and its parts. *Annual Review of Anthropology, 29*(1): 287–328.

Shim, J. K., Bentz, M., Vasquez, E., Jeske, M., Saperstein, A., Fullerton, S. M., Foti, N., McMahon, C., and Lee, S. S. J. (2022). Strategies of inclusion: The tradeoffs of pursuing "baked in" diversity through place-based recruitment. *Social Science and Medicine, 306*: 115132.

Simon, H. A. (1997). *Models of bounded rationality: Empirically grounded economic reason* (Vol. 3). MIT Press, Cambridge.

Skorburg, J. A., O'Doherty, K., and Friesen, P. (2024). Persons or data points? Ethics, artificial intelligence, and the participatory turn in mental health research. *American Psychologist, 79*(1): 137.

Sleeboom-Faulkner, M., Chekar, C. K., Faulkner, A., Heitmeyer, C., Marouda, M., Rosemann, A., Chaisinthop, N., Chang, H. C. J., Ely, A., Kato, M., and Patra, P. K. (2016). Comparing national home-keeping and the regulation of translational stem cell applications: An international perspective. *Social Science and Medicine, 153*: 240–249.

Sleeboom-Faulkner, M. E. (2016). The large grey area between 'bona fide' and 'rogue' stem cell interventions—Ethical acceptability and the need to include local variability. *Technological Forecasting and Social Change, 109*: 76–86.

Slota, S. C., & Bowker, G. C. (2017). How infrastructures matter. *The Handbook of Science and Technology Studies, 4*, 529–554.

Smith, R., and Hoppe, R. (1991). The patient's story: Integrating the patient- and physician-centered approaches to interviewing. *Annals of International Medicine, 115*: 470e7.

Spanish Presidency Council of Europe. (2023). MareNostrum5 opening. Available at https://mn5-opening.bsc.es/

Stalla-Bourdillon, S. (2023). The definition of "anonymization" is changing in the EU: Here's what that means. *The International Association of Privacy Professionals (IAPP).* Available at https://iapp.org/news/a/the-definition-of-anonymization-is-changing-in-the-eu-heres-what-that-means

Star, S. L. (1999). The ethnography of infrastructure. *American Behavioral Scientist, 43*(3): 377–391.

Star, S. L., and Ruhleder, K. (1994). Steps towards an ecology of infrastructure: Complex problems in design and access for large-scale collaborative systems. *Proceedings of the 1994 ACM conference on computer supported cooperative work*, Chapel Hill North Carolina USA: 253–264.

Stark, L., and Hutson, J. (2021). Physiognomic artificial intelligence. *Fordham Intellectual Property, Media and Entertainment Law Journal, 32*: 922.

Statista. (2018). Willingness to wear health tracking technology U. S. Percentage of U. S. adults that were willing to wear technology that tracks select health statistics as of 2018. *Statista.* Available at https://www.statista.com/statistics/829479/willingness-to-wear-health-tracking-technology-us-adults.

Steinsbekk, K. S., Kåre Myskja, B., and Solberg, B. (2013). Broad consent versus dynamic consent in biobank research: Is passive participation an ethical problem? *European Journal of Human Genetics, 21*(9): 897–902.

Stewart, C. (2025). Willingness to wear health tracking technology U. S. Percentage of U. S. adults that were willing to wear technology that tracks select health statistics as of 2018. Statista. Available at https://www.statista.com/statistics/829479/willingness-to-wear-health-tracking-technology-us-adults.

Stewart, M. (2001). Towards a global definition of patient centred care: The patient should be the judge of patient centred care. *British Medical Journal, 322*(7284): 444–445.

Stilgoe, J, Owen, R, and Macnaghten, P. (2013). Developing a framework for responsible innovation. *Research Policy, 42*: 1568–1580.

Stivers, T., and Timmermans, S. (2017). The actionability of exome sequencing testing results. *Sociology of Health Illness, 39*: 1542–1556.

Strimbu, K., and Tavel, J. A. (2010). What are biomarkers? *Current Opinion in HIV and AIDS, 5*(6): 463–466.

Sun, S., and Ching, A. H. (2021). Social systems matter: Precision medicine, public health, and the medical model. *East Asian Science, Technology and Society: An International Journal, 15*(4): 439–466.

Sun, S., and Ong, Z. (2024). *The color of precision medicine*. Routledge, London.

Superchi, C., Bouvier, F. B., Gerardi, C., Carmona, M., San Miguel, L., Sánchez-Gómez, L. M., Imaz-Iglesia, I., Garcia, P., Demotes, J., Banzi, R., and Porcher, R. (2022). Study designs for clinical trials applied to personalised medicine: A scoping review. *British Medical Journal (BMJ) Open, 12*(5): e052926.

Surendra, H. M. H. S., and Mohan, H. S. (2017). A review of synthetic data generation methods for privacy preserving data publishing. *International Journal of Scientific and Technology Research, 6*(3): 95–101.

Swaminathan, S., Pécoul, B., Abdullah, H., Christou, C., Gray, G., IJsselmuiden, C., Kieny, M. P., Mazzucato, M., von Messling, V., Ogutu, B., and Reeder, J. (2022). Reboot biomedical RandD in the global public interest. *Nature, 602*(7896): 207–210.

Swan, M. (2013). The quantified self: Fundamental disruption in big data science and biological discovery. *Big Data, 2*(1): 85–98.

Swan, M. (2012). Health (2050): The realization of personalized medicine through crowdsourcing, the quantified self, and the participatory biocitizen. *Journal of Personalized Medicine, 2*: 93–118.

Takahashi, K., and Yamanaka, S. (2006). Induction of pluripotent stem cells from mouse embryonic and adult fibroblast cultures by defined factors. *Cell, 126*(4): 663–676.

Takashima, K., Morrison, M., and Minari, J. (2021). Reflection on the enactment and impact of safety laws for regenerative medicine in Japan. *Stem Cell Reports, 16*(6): 1425–1434.

TallBear, K. (2013). Genomic articulations of indigeneity. *Social Studies of Science, 43*(4): 509–533.

Tanner, J. M. (1981). *A history of the study of human growth.* Cambridge University Press, Cambridge.

Tarantino, P., Mazzarella, L., Marra, A., Trapani, D., and Curigliano, G. (2021). The evolving paradigm of biomarker actionability: Histology-agnosticism as a spectrum, rather than a binary quality. *Cancer Treatment Review, 94*: 102169.

Tarkkala, H., Helén, I., and Snell, K. (2019). From health to wealth: The future of personalized medicine in the making. *Futures, 109*: 142–152.

Tarran, B. (2016). Deep concerns over DeepMind's access to patient data. *Significance, 13*(3): 4–5.

Tattersall, R. (1996). A history of growth hormone. *Hormone Research, 46*(4–5): 236–247.

Taylor-Gooby, P. (2006). Social divisions of trust: Scepticism and democracy in the GM Nation? debate. *Journal of Risk Research, 9*(1): 75–95.

Teare, H. J., Hogg, J., Kaye, J., Luqmani, R., Rush, E., Turner, A., Watts, L., Williams, M., and Javaid, M. K. (2017). The RUDY study: Using digital technologies to enable a research partnership. *European Journal of Human Genetics, 25*(7): 816–822.

Teare, H. J., Morrison, M., Whitley, E. A., and Kaye, J. (2015). Towards 'Engagement 2.0': Insights from a study of dynamic consent with biobank participants. *Digit Health, 1*: 1–13.

Teare, H. J. A., Prictor, M., and Kaye, J. (2021). Reflections on dynamic consent in biomedical research: The story so far. *European Journal of Human Genetics, 29*: 649–656.

Tempini, N., and Leonelli, S. (2021). Actionable data for precision oncology: Framing trustworthy evidence for exploratory research and clinical diagnostics. *Social Science and Medicine, 272*: 113760.

Ten Have, H. A. (2001). Genetics and culture: The geneticization thesis. *Medicine, Health Care and Philosophy, 4*: 295–304.

Terlizzi, V., and Farrell, P. M. (2024). Update on advances in cystic fibrosis towards a cure and implications for primary care clinicians. *Current Problems in Pediatric and Adolescent Health Care, 54*(6): 101637.

Terry, S. F., Terry, P. F., Rauen, K. A., Uitto, J., and Bercovitch, L. G. (2007). Advocacy groups as research organizations: The PXE International example. *Nature Reviews Genetics, 8*(2): 157–164.

Thaler, R. (1980). Toward a positive theory of consumer choice. *Journal of Economic Behavior and Organization, 1*(1): 39–60.

Timmermans, S., and Buchbinder, M. (2010). Patients-in-waiting: Living between sickness and health in the genomics era. *Journal of Health and Social Behavior, 51*(4): 408–423.

Timmermans, S., and Epstein, S. (2010). A world of standards but not a standard world: Toward a sociology of standards and standardization. *Annual Review of Sociology, 36*(1): 69–89.

Tironi, M., and Valderrama, M. (2021). Experimenting with the social life of homes: Sensor governmentality and its frictions. *Science as Culture, 30*: 192–215.

Torreele, E., Mazzucato, M., and Li, H. L. (2021). *Delivering the people's vaccine.* UCL Institute for Innovation and Public Purpose, London.

Townsend, M. (2017, 19 August). Home office used charity data map to deport rough sleepers. *The Observer*. Available at https://okwd.uk/pt4

Trias, E., Juan, M., Urbano-Ispizua, A., and Calvo, G. (2022). The hospital exemption pathway for the approval of advanced therapy medicinal products: An underused opportunity? The case of the CAR-T ARI-0001. *Bone Marrow Transplantation, 57*(2): 156–159.

Tsing, A. (2012). On Nonscalability: The living world is not amenable to precision-nested scales. *Common Knowledge, 18*(3): 505–524.

Turner, B. S. (1995). *Medical power and social knowledge* (2nd edition). Sage, London.

Turner, L., and Knoepfler, P. (2016). Selling stem cells in the USA: Assessing the direct-to-consumer industry. *Cell Stem Cell, 19*(2): 154–157.

Tutton, R. (2014). *Genomics and the reimagining of personalised medicine*. Ashgate, Farnham.

Tutton, R., and Prainsack, B. (2011). Enterprising or altruistic selves? Making up research subjects in genetics research. *Sociology of Health and Illness, 33*(7): 1081–1095.

Tutton, R., Smart, A., Martin, P. A., Ashcroft, R., and Ellison, G. (2008). Genotyping the future: Scientists' expectations about race/ethnicity after BiDil. *Journal of Law Medicine and Ethics, 36*(3): 464–470.

Umemura, M. (2019). Challenging the problem of 'fit': Advancing the regenerative medicine industries in the United States, Britain and Japan. *The Business of Health, 61*(3): 456–480.

Umemura, M., and Morrison, M. (2021). Comparative lessons in regenerative medicine readiness: Learning from the UK and Japanese experience. *Regenerative Medicine, 16*(3): 269–282.

Van Aken, J., Schmedders, M., Feuerstein, G., and Kolleck, R. (2003). Prospects and limits of pharmacogenetics: The Thiopurine Methyl Transferase (TPMT) experience. *American Journal of Pharmacogenomics, 3*(3): 149–155.

Van Cutsem, E., Köhne, C. H., Hitre, E., Zaluski, J., Chang Chien, C. R., Makhson, A., D'Haens, G., Pintér, T., Lim, R., Bodoky, G., and Roh, J. K. (2009). Cetuximab and chemotherapy as initial treatment for metastatic colorectal cancer. *New England Journal of Medicine, 360*(14): 1408–1417.

Van Dijck, J., Nieborg, D., & Poell, T. (2019). Reframing platform power. *Internet Policy Review, 8*(2): 1–18.

Van Hoyweghen, I., and Aarden, E. (2022). One for all, all for one? Containing the promise of solidarity in precision medicine. *Critical Public Health, 32*(4): 568–579.

Van Lente, H. (1993). *Promising technology: The dynamics of expectations in technological developments.* Proefschrift Universiteit Twente, Enschede.

Van Lente, H., Spitters, C., and Peine, A. (2013). Comparing technological hype cycles: Towards a theory. *Technological Forecasting and Social Change, 80*: 1615–1628.

Vaught, J. B., & Henderson, M. K. (2011). Biological sample collection, processing, storage and information management. *International Agency For Research On Cancer (IARC) Scientific Publications, 163*(163): 23–42.

Verbelen, M., Weale, M. E., and Lewis, C. M. (2017). Cost-effectiveness of pharmacogenetic-guided treatment: Are we there yet? *The Pharmacogenomics Journal, 17*: 395–402.

Vermeulen, N., Haddow, G., Seymour, T., Faulkner-Jones, A., and Shu, W. (2017). 3D bioprint me: A socioethical view of bioprinting human organs and tissues. *Journal of Medical Ethics, 43*(9): 618–624.

Vezyridis, P., and Timmons, S. (2016). Dissenting from Care.data: An analysis of opt-out forms. *Journal of Medical Ethics, 42*(12): 792–796.

Vincent, J. (2022). *Beyond measure: The hidden history of measurement from cubits to quantum constants.* W. W. Norton, New York.

Vincent, J. A. (2006). Ageing contested: Anti-ageing science and the cultural construction of old age. *Sociology, 40*(4): 681–698.

Wadmann, S., and Hauge, A. M. (2020). Strategies of stratification: Regulating market access in the era of personalized medicine. *Social Studies of Science, 51*(4): 628–653.

Wadmann, S., Hauge, A. M., and Navne, L. E. (2023). Good conduct in a context of rationing: A case study of how frontline professionals deal with distributive dilemmas of novel gene therapies. *Sociology of Health and Illness, 45*(3): 684–704.

Wadmann, S., Johansen, A. B., Born, A. P., & Kessel, L. (2024). Infrastructuring precision medicine: Making gene therapies for rare diseases workable in practice. *Social Science & Medicine, 351*, 116966.

Wainwright, S. P., Michael, M., and Williams, C. (2008). Shifting paradigms? Reflections on regenerative medicine, embryonic stem cells and pharmaceuticals. *Sociology of Health and Illness, 30*(6): 959–974.

Waldby, C., and Salter, B. (2008). Global governance in human embryonic stem cell science: Standardisation and bioethics in research and patenting. *Studies in Ethics, Law, and Technology, 2*(1), 1–23.

Walsh, K., Wallace, A., Pavis, M., Olszowy, N., Griffin, J., and Hawkins, N. (2021). Intellectual property rights and access in crisis. *IIC-International Review of Intellectual Property and Competition Law, 52*(4): 379–416.

Wan, Z., Hazel, J. W., Clayton, E. W., Vorobeychik, Y., Kantarcioglu, M., and Malin, B. A. (2022). Sociotechnical safeguards for genomic data privacy. *Nature Reviews Genetics, 23*(7): 429–445.

Webster, A., and Eriksson, L. (2008). Governance-by-standards in the field of stem cells: Managing uncertainty in the world of "basic innovation". *New Genetics and Society, 27*(2): 99–111.

Webster, A., and Gardner, J. (2019). Aligning technology and institutional readiness: The adoption of innovation. *Technology Analysis and Strategic Management, 31*(10): 1229–1241.

Webster, A., Haddad, C., and Waldby, C. (2011). Experimental heterogeneity and standardisation: Stem cell products and the clinical trial process. *BioSocieties, 6*: 401–419.

Welsh, I., and Wynne, B. (2013). Science, scientism, and imaginaries of publics in the UK: Passive objects, incipient threats. *Science as Culture, 22*(4): 540–566.

Whitney, C. D., and Norman, J. (2024, June). Real risks of fake data: Synthetic data, diversity-washing and consent circumvention. *Proceedings of the 2024 ACM conference on fairness, accountability, and transparency*, Rio de Janeiro Brazil: 1733–1744.

Wired.com. (N.D.). Wired insider: How personalised medicine is changing healthcare. *Wired.* Available at https://www.wired.com/sponsored/story/personalised-medicine-changing-healthcare/

WMA. (2002). Declaration of Taipei. Research on health databases, big data and biobanks. *World Medical Association.* Available at https://www.wma.net/policies-post/wma-declaration-of-taipei-on-ethical-considerations-regarding-health-databases-and-biobanks/

WMA. (1964). Declaration of Helsinki – Ethical principles for medical research involving human subjects. *World Medical Association.* Available at https://www.wma.net/policies-post/wma-declaration-of-helsinki/

Wolf, G. (2010). The data-driven life. *The New York Times.* Available at https://www.nytimes.com/2010/05/02/magazine/02self-measurement-t.html

Wynne, B. (2002). Risk and environment as legitimatory discourses of technology: Reflexivity inside out? *Current Sociology, 50*: 459–477.

Zanatta, R. A. (2023). A proteção coletiva dos dados pessoais no Brasil: A defesa de direitos entre autoritarismo e democracia. Doctoral Thesis, Universidade de São Paulo, Brazil. Available at https://www.teses.usp.br/teses/disponiveis/106/106132/tde-12062023-153956/publico/TeseZANATTA.pdf

INDEX

Note: Page numbers followed by "n" denote endnotes.